# ANOTHER WEIGHTLOSS GIMMICK? MAYBE NOT

# ANOTHER WEIGHTLOSS GIMMICK? MAYBE NOT

## Eliminate Blue Light – Maximize Melatonin – Develop Brown Fat – Burn White Fat.

RICHARD L. HANSLER, PHD

ISBN-10: 1494404184
ISBN-13: 9781494404185

Library of Congress Control Number: 2013922843
CreateSpace Independent Publishing Platform,
North Charleston, South Carolina

# ACKNOWLEDGMENTS

First, I must acknowledge my wife, Wanda, for her understanding and patience with me as I try to pursue my desire to help people by letting them know about the dangers that lie in an ordinary light bulb. I thank her for that support. I want to thank my son-in-law, Mark Thomsen, for the attractive design of the cover for this book. I also want to thank the partners in Photonic Developments LLC who sponsor the website where low-blue-light products are available www.lowbluelights.com. They are Dr. Edward Carome, Dr. Martin Alpert, and Vilnis Kubulins. Together, we are building a business based on trying to help people to better health. I also want to thank Dan Carome, our customer service person, for the great job he does in keeping our customers happy but also for his very valuable contribution in producing new products like the filters for large flat-screen TVs and computers and for mobile devices. I also want to thank the people at CreateSpace for making publishing this book a pleasure.

# TABLE OF CONTENTS

# PREFACE

I did research for GE Lighting for more than forty years and helped develop new, more efficient and brighter light bulbs. After retiring from GE, in 1996, I came to John Carroll University, where I founded the Lighting Innovations Institute. In the institute, we develop new lighting systems for customers, including NASA, the FAA, and commercial companies that provide airfield lighting. We were asked by one of our customers to develop an LED source to treat people with seasonal affective disorder (SAD). That got me interested in how light affects health, and I was shocked to learn that people who were exposed to light at night (shift-work nurses) had about double the incidence of breast cancer as nurses who did not work nights. I learned that using ordinary light during the night, when the body should be producing melatonin, increased the risk for diabetes, *obesity*, heart disease, breast cancer, colon cancer, and prostate cancer. I learned that it is primarily the blue rays in ordinary white light that cause melatonin suppression. Learning this, my team in the institute—Dr. Edward Carome, Vilnis Kubulins, and I—developed light bulbs that don't make blue light and eyeglasses that eliminate the blue rays. We formed a company, Photonic Developments LLC and opened a website where these products are available at www.lowbluelights.com. I wrote three books *Great Sleep! Reduced Cancer!*, *Heroes of Cancer Prevention Research*, and *Pregnant? New Baby? Need Sleep!* They are available on the website or as Kindle books for ninety-nine cents each. That's the history so far. Now, I'm faced with a new task.

How do you start a book that tries to help people who are interested in avoiding becoming obese or who are already overweight or obese? It isn't obvious, at least not to me. I've been studying the effect that light has on sleep and health for more than ten years. We know we are helping thousands of people sleep better, and more and more people are learning about how that works. But right now, we want to extend that to helping people control their weight. I need to explain how that works as simply as we explain how wearing glasses that block blue light for a few hours before bedtime helps people sleep better. In that case, it only requires explaining that exposing the eyes to ordinary light during the evening stops the pineal gland from making melatonin, the sleep hormone. It's actually the blue rays in ordinary light that cause suppression of melatonin. Wearing glasses that block the blue rays allows the pineal gland to make melatonin. By bedtime, there is plenty present in the bloodstream so it's easy to fall asleep and the sleep is deeper and more refreshing. How that same action of avoiding blue light before bedtime helps people control their weight is a little more complicated. For one thing, you need to do this at the same time every evening. I guess I need to start by explaining why sleep is so important for weight control.

# INTRODUCTION

The number of people who are overweight or obese has reached record levels, and obesity is regarded as the most significant health problem worldwide. There is no quick solution to this problem, but one factor that has been ignored up to now is the effect that reduced time spent sleeping may have on weight gain. One result of less time sleeping is less time in darkness. That results in a reduction of the amount of melatonin produced by the body. Correcting that situation is the focus of this book, which offers a dramatically different approach to controlling weight. Some are calling it the "brown fat revolution."

# CHAPTER 1
## Why and How to Fix Your Sleep

People used to say "Everyone knows sleep is important." That doesn't seem to be the case anymore. For some people, sleep has become what they do when they have nothing more important to do. Average sleep duration has dropped dramatically over the last twenty years. So the first thing you may want to consider doing to control your weight is to rethink your attitude toward sleep.

To give you something to ponder, consider how scientists regard sleep as it relates to being overweight and obese. On the US government website www.pubmed.gov, one can put in search words and come up with abstracts of the studies published in technical journals. If one searches using "obesity" and "sleep," one finds an astonishing 5,876 abstracts, and if one adds 2013 (the year this is being written), one still finds 590 studies published this year on the relationship between sleep and obesity. That's almost two a day. We will be looking at quite a few of those studies in the last half of this book, but for now, we will only mention this as a way of helping you appreciate that sleep is indeed important when you are serious about controlling your weight.

Over the millions of years humans have evolved in the parts of the world near the equator, there were twelve hours of light and twelve hours of darkness. People most likely slept much of those twelve hours of darkness. Moonlight was very likely more highly appreciated than it is today. Even after fire was discovered and candles and oil lamps became available, most people were probably too poor to use them often. Much of the long, dark nights were spent sleeping.

It is only within the last one hundred years or so that we have had reliable, bright artificial light. It is for a considerably shorter time that we have had portable electronic devices with bright screens that we can even take to bed with us. This explosion in the time when we are exposed to light has had a profound effect on our sleeping habits. Most people in the developed counties of the world have considerably less than eight hours of sleep, and many have less than six hours a night.

The major conclusion of all the studies of sleep and obesity is that those who sleep seven or eight hours a night are much less likely to become overweight or obese than those who sleep less than seven hours a night. Theories of why this is true include that the extra hours of wakefulness allow more time for eating. A different theory, to which I subscribe, is that the exposure to light while awake prevents the body from producing melatonin. The fact that exposing the eyes to light stops the flow of melatonin from the pineal gland was discovered very early, but it wasn't until 2001 that it was learned that it is primarily the blue rays in ordinary white light that stop the production of melatonin. Unfortunately, the most recent types of light bulbs produce significantly more of the blue rays than the incandescent lamp (gradually being made illegal). The bright screens of smartphones, tablets, and TVs all produce large amounts of blue light.

This lack of melatonin as a result of exposure to light in the hours before bedtime results in difficulty in falling asleep, an increase in the time to reach deep sleep, and, consequently, less time spent in deep sleep. This lack of melatonin is also thought to increase the risk of a number of diseases, including obesity, diabetes, heart disease, and breast and prostate cancer.

Having spent more than forty years doing research for GE Lighting on better and brighter light bulbs, I felt that I had a responsibility to do something about this damaging effect of using light at night. The discovery that it was the blue rays in ordinary white light that was doing the damage offers a way to solve this problem.

As I mentioned in the foreword, my small group of physicists at John Carroll University developed light bulbs that don't make blue light. We also developed eyeglasses that eliminate the blue rays. We formed a small company, Photonic Developments LLC, which created a website in 2005 at www.lowbluelights.com that sells these products. The glasses are sold with a money-back guarantee if they don't improve sleep. They help about

90 percent of those who try them. Some people make almost no melatonin even in total darkness. They will not be helped by using our glasses.

That the glasses do work was established by an experiment at the University of Toronto in 2005 in which the subjects in the experiment worked under bright lights while wearing glasses that blocked the blue light. Their melatonin was sampled throughout the night. It was found they produced melatonin just as they had on an earlier night when they were in darkness. The glasses block all the light at wavelengths less than about 530 nanometers (blue-green).

To get the full benefit of using these products both for great sleep and reduced risk of various diseases, I recommend the following steps.

1. Get up at about the same time every morning and expose your eyes to lots of light. Wash in a brightly lit bathroom. Have breakfast in a brightly lit kitchen. Walk outside for a few minutes.

2. Put on low-blue-light glasses about twelve or thirteen hours after the time you got up. Wear them until you are in your dark bedroom. You may also use low-blue-light light bulbs and filters on electronic devices instead.

This doesn't work during the summer when it's light until ten o'clock. If you find you get too sleepy too soon, put on your glasses a little later.

3.  Go to bed at about the same time every night.

4.  If you need to get up during the night, do not expose your eyes to ordinary white light. Use a low-blue-light night-light. If you have to turn on a light, make sure you have your glasses on or use a low-blue-light light bulb.

If you find you can't do all this without exception, don't worry about it. Once you have your daily rhythm of light and dark very well established, missing out for a day or two now and then will not have much effect. We know from the experience of jet lag that it is not easy to shift our daily schedule (also called circadian rhythm). It may take two or three days to get used to daylight saving time changes.

You may be thinking to yourself, *How big a deal is sleep? The connection between sleep and being fat might be just because fat people have trouble breathing when they lie down so they don't sleep much.* That is true, and many overweight people suffer from sleep apnea, which can kill them if sufficiently serious and untreated. However, studies in which people are followed for long periods have shown that those who sleep less are more likely to become obese than those who sleep seven or eight hours a night.

A study of studies found for a sample of 30,000 children and 604,000 adults that for children the odds ratio (OR) for short sleepers becoming obese was 1.89 and for adults the OR was 1.55. This means that if you select equal numbers of short sleepers and normal sleepers, for every one hundred of the normal sleepers who become obese there will be 189 short sleepers who become obese. Putting it another way, if you are a short-sleeping child, your chance of becoming obese is almost double that of a child who sleeps seven or eight hours or more a night.

There is another problem besides losing melatonin when you expose your eyes to light during the time when melatonin is (or should be) flowing. It's referred to as "disruption of the circadian cycle." Living things have built-in clocks. These internal or circadian clocks are controlled by light. When we go from darkness to light in the morning, it resets the clock. Twelve hours later, the pineal gland is signaled by the clock to begin making melatonin. The amount in the blood builds to a maximum about six hours later and drops to near zero about the time we go from dark to light, and it starts all over again. This is the way it worked during the millions of years we were evolving.

Humans evolved near the equator where it's light for twelve hours and dark for twelve hours year-round. When humans moved north and south, away from the equator, the hours of light and dark changed with the seasons. Animals' circadian clocks developed into calendars as well as clocks. This allows the arctic fox to turn white in advance of winter and brown in advance of summer and allows sheep to conceive lambs in the fall to be born in the spring. It also results in humans living in Alaska having serious problems sleeping. Maintaining a solid circadian cycle isn't easy when it's light all night in the summer and dark all day in the winter. Low-blue-light products are very helpful during the summer as are ordinary white light sources to be used during the winter "days" when it's continuously dark outside.

Most of the world's population does not live under such extreme conditions but does experience the changes with the seasons. By controlling light using glasses and light bulbs, a stable circadian cycle can be maintained throughout the year. Opaque shades in the bedroom may also be helpful. The eyelids only transmit about 3 percent of white light. Since the transmitted light is red (blood in the eyelids), it is unlikely the early morning light will suppress melatonin if one is sleeping in a room without shades during the summer.

Probably the main source of disruption of the circadian cycle is having to get up at night. For most young adults, this is not a problem. However, when a woman becomes pregnant, she is likely to need to get up frequently during the night. If she turns on an ordinary light, it will disrupt the setting of her internal clock so her normal flow of melatonin may not begin at the usual time.

Using light bulbs that don't produce blue light or putting on amber glasses becomes important.

When the baby arrives, getting up many times during the night becomes the normal routine for both the mother and father. The blue-blocking glasses and low-blue-light light bulbs are vital. For the sake of the baby, low blue lighting in the nursery is important. During pregnancy, the baby's circadian rhythm will be in synchrony with the mother's since melatonin flows easily across the placental barrier. This will continue if the mother is breastfeeding since her melatonin will occur in her milk at the same time as in her blood. Maintaining a strong circadian rhythm of getting up and exposing the eyes to light in the morning and avoiding ordinary white light in the evening and of eating and sleeping will go a long way toward preventing adding extra weight while pregnant. It will also assist in losing any extra weight put on during pregnancy.

Shift work is another situation in which the dual problem of loss of melatonin and disruption of the circadian rhythm make sleep difficult. Use of the amber glasses that block blue light may be of value to those working night or rotating shifts. Permanent night-shift workers should try to turn their days into nights with blackout shades. My recommendation is the same as for everyone else. They should put on the glasses two or three hours before going to bed in darkness during the day. They should keep the same schedule on days off and weekends. This should maximize their production of melatonin and thus help them avoid any sleep problems.

For rotating shift workers on slowly rotating shifts (e.g., monthly), the best plan is to try to adapt as the shifts rotate and use the glasses two or three hours ahead of bedtime regardless of which shift they are on. Again, they should sleep in darkness.

For quickly rotating shift workers (a week or less), it may be possible to keep the body on the same schedule as when they are working days. That is, put on the glasses at the same time every evening (e.g., 8:00 p.m.) whether planning to go to bed or to work at 11:00. Wear them until bedtime on days off or all night while working (e.g., until 7:00 a.m.). Since melatonin will be present while at work, sleepiness is potentially a problem. One brief study by Kayumov at the University of Toronto found no decline in performance under these conditions, i.e., while wearing amber glasses while working at night.[1]

---

[1] J Clin Endocrinol Metab. 2005 May;90(5):2755-61. Epub 2005 Feb 15.
**Blocking low-wavelength light prevents nocturnal melatonin suppression with no adverse effect on performance during simulated shift work.**
Kayumov L, Casper RF, Hawa RJ, Perelman B, Chung SA, Sokalsky S, Shapiro CM.

# CHAPTER 2
## White and Brown Fat

*For much of this chapter, we rely on writings from the popular literature, websites, blogs, and ads.*

Searched the Mayo Clinic website: www.mayoclinic.org for "brown fat"

How is brown fat different from other fat?

What is brown fat? How is it different from other body fat?

Answer from Donald Hensrud, MD

Brown fat, also called brown adipose tissue, is a special type of body fat that is turned on, or activated, when you get cold. Brown fat produces heat to help maintain your body temperature in cold conditions.

Brown fat has generated interest among doctors and researchers for some time because it appears to be able to use regular body fat as fuel. And equally promising, it looks as if exercise may stimulate hormones that activate brown fat.

Researchers are looking at whether brown fat's calorie-burning properties can be harnessed for weight loss. It's too soon to know whether these efforts will pay off. In the meantime, be sure to include physical activity in your weight management plans.

To say that brown fat has generated interest among doctors is a huge understatement. Brown fat is a hot item, at least among researchers. Searching in PubMed with just "brown fat" turns up 9,887 abstracts of technical papers. Of these, roughly 10 percent were published within the past year.

One of the strongest arguments that sleep, darkness, and/or melatonin may be the key(s) to avoiding obesity is the observed change in body fat in small animals like the Syrian hamster during the changing seasons[1].

Melatonin has been shown not only to stimulate the transition of white fat to brown fat but also to stimulate the conversion of brown fat to heat.

Chronodisruption is another concept that has been shown to have a strong relationship to obesity. It refers to interruption of the normal circadian rhythm, such as brought about by jet lag, shift work, light at night, and social jet lag (staying up late on Saturday night).

One piece of evidence pointing to the importance of brown fat is the observation that the fraction of fat that is brown fat is highest in lean individuals.

Most recent studies report a third type of fat cell (brite / beige) that is found within the white fat. Its origin is different, but its action is the same as regular brown fat.

A good introduction to the importance of brown fat for weight control is in the following discussion from the National Institutes of Health *Director's Blog* entry: "Brown Fat, White Fat, Good Fat, Bad Fat" by Dr. Francis Collins[2]:

> Fat has been villainized; but all fat was not created equal. Our two main types of fat—brown and white—play different roles. Now, two teams of NIH-funded researchers have enriched our understanding of adipose tissue. The first team discovered the genetic switch that triggers the development of brown fat [1], and the second figured out how the body can recruit white fat and transform it into brown [2].

---

[2]  Posted March 26, 2013.

Why would we want to change white fat into brown? White fat stores energy as large fat droplets, while brown fat has much smaller droplets and is specialized to burn them, yielding heat. Brown fat cells are packed with energy generating powerhouses called mitochondria that contain iron—which gives them their brown color. Infants are born with rich stores of brown fat (about 5% of total body mass) on the upper spine and shoulders to keep them warm. It used to be thought that brown fat disappeared by adulthood—but it turns out we harbor small reserves in our shoulders and neck.

In mice, brown fat does something remarkable: it burns more calories when mice are overfed, protecting them from obesity. (Don't you wish eating a plate of fries did that for you?) Furthermore, mice genetically predisposed to have with [sic] extra brown fat are actually leaner and healthier. In humans, there is evidence that more brown fat is associated with a lower body weight. So, how might we increase our brown fat production?

The team led by the University of Pennsylvania figured out the switch for creating a brown fat cell—a protein called early B cell factor-2 (Ebf2). Comparing the active genes in brown and white fat cells, they discovered Ebf2 is present in larger quantities in brown fat. This protein seems to mark which genes will later be turned on to transform certain types of precursor cells into brown fat. When the team engineered mice lacking this protein, the animals had white fat cells on their upper back and spine rather than the typical brown. When the team expressed high levels of Ebf2 in white fat, these cells turned brown and consumed more oxygen—a sign they were producing more heat.

The second team, led by Harvard's Joslin Diabetes Center, noted that mice have two types of brown fat: constitutive brown fat, which they have from birth, and "recruitable" brown fat, scattered throughout the muscles and white fat. When researchers engineered mice lacking a protein called Type 1A BMP-receptor (BMPR1A)—which is needed for the correct development of brown fat—the mice were born with just a tiny bit of constitutive brown fat on their back.

You would think that these mice would be terribly cold. Surprisingly, they kept a normal body temperature. How did they manage this feat?

The lack of brown fat apparently sends a signal via the brain to the recruitable fat cells, telling them to make the switch and transform into brown fat. The mice stayed warm, and the recruited brown fat even protected them from obesity.

In humans, too much abdominal white fat promotes heart disease, diabetes, and many other metabolic diseases. It would be potentially therapeutic if we could transform some of our white fat into brown. Determining which genes control the development of white and brown fat may be the first step toward developing game changing treatments for diabetes and obesity.

## References:

[1] EBF2 determines and maintains brown adipocyte identity. Rajakumari S, Wu J, Ishibashi J, Lim HW, Giang AH, Won KJ, Reed RR, Seale P. *Cell Metab.* 2013 Mar 12
[2] Brown-fat paucity due to impaired BMP signaling induces compensatory browning of white fat. Schulz TJ, Huang P, Huang TL, Xue R, McDougall LE, Townsend KL, Cypess AM, Mishina Y, Gussoni E, Tseng YH. *Nature.* 2013 Mar 13

*NIH support: the National Institute of Diabetes and Digestive and Kidney Diseases; and the National Institute of General Medical Sciences*

The following article explains more about the distribution of fat in the body.

From the WebMD Feature Archive:

**Everything You Need to Know about Fat, Including an Explanation of which Is Worse—Belly Fat or Thigh Fat**

By Kathleen Doheny

WebMD Feature

Reviewed by Louise Chang, MD

For most of us, body fat has a bad reputation. From the dimply stuff that plagues women's thighs to the beer bellies that can pop out in middle-aged men, fat is typically something we agonize over, scorn, and try to exercise away.

But for scientists, fat is intriguing—and becoming more so every day. "Fat is one of the most fascinating organs out there," says Aaron Cypess, MD, PhD, an instructor of medicine at Harvard Medical School and a research associate at the Joslin Diabetes Center in Boston. "We are only now beginning to understand fat."

"Fat has more functions in the body than we thought," agrees Rachel Whitmer, PhD, research scientist at the Kaiser Permanente Division of Research in Oakland, Calif., who has studied the links between fat and brain health.

To get the skinny on fat, WebMD asked four experts on fat—who, not surprisingly, prefer not to be called fat experts—to fill us in.

Fat is known to have two main purposes, says Susan Fried, PhD, director of the Boston Obesity and Nutrition Research Center at Boston University and a long-time researcher in the field.

- Fat stores excess calories in a safe way so you can mobilize the fat stores when you're hungry.

- Fat releases hormones that control metabolism.

But that's the broad brushstroke picture. Read on for details about various types of fat—brown, white, subcutaneous, visceral, and belly fat.

## Brown Fat

Brown fat has gotten a lot of buzz recently, with the discovery that it's not the mostly worthless fat scientists had thought.

In recent studies, scientists have found that lean people tend to have more brown fat than overweight or obese people—and that when stimulated it can burn calories. Scientists are eyeing it as a potential obesity treatment if they can figure out a way to increase a person's brown fat or stimulate existing brown fat.

It's known that children have more brown fat than adults, and it's what helps them keep warm. Brown fat stores decline in adults but still help with warmth. "We've shown brown fat is more active in people in Boston in colder months," Cypess says, leading to the idea of sleeping in chillier rooms to burn a few more calories.

Brown fat is now thought to be more like muscle than like white fat. When activated, brown fat burns white fat.

Although leaner adults have more brown fat than heavier people, even their brown fat cells are greatly outnumbered by white fat cells. "A 150-pound person might have 20 or 30 pounds of fat," Cypess says. "They are only going to have 2 or 3 ounces of brown fat."

But that 2 ounces, he says, if maximally stimulated, could burn off 300 to 500 calories a day—enough to lose up to a pound in a week.

"You might give people a drug that increases brown fat," he says. "We're working on one."

But even if the drug to stimulate brown fat pans out, Cypess warns, it won't be a cure-all for weight issues. It may, however, help a person achieve more weight loss combined with a sound diet and exercise regimen.

## White Fat

White fat is much more plentiful than brown, experts agree. The job of white fat is to store energy and produce hormones that are then secreted into the bloodstream.

Small fat cells produce a "good guy" hormone called adiponectin, which makes the liver and muscles sensitive to the hormone insulin, in the process making us less susceptible to diabetes and heart disease.

When people become fat, the production of adiponectin slows down or shuts down, setting them up for disease, according to Fried and others.

## Subcutaneous Fat

Subcutaneous fat is found directly under the skin. It's the fat that's measured using skin-fold calipers to estimate your total body fat.

In terms of overall health, subcutaneous fat in the thighs and buttocks, for instance, may not be as bad and may have some potential benefits, says Cypess. "It may not cause as many problems" as other types of fat, specifically the deeper, visceral fat, he says.

But subcutaneous fat cells on the belly may be another story, says Fried. There's emerging evidence that the danger of big bellies lies not only in the deep visceral fat but also the subcutaneous fat.

## Visceral Fat

Visceral or "deep" fat wraps around the inner organs and spells trouble for your health. How do you know if you have it? "If you have a large waist or belly, of course you have visceral fat," Whitmer says. Visceral fat drives up your risk for diabetes, heart disease, stroke, and even dementia.

Visceral fat is thought to play a larger role in insulin resistance—which boosts risk of diabetes—than other fat, Whitmer tells WebMD. It's not clear why, but it could explain or partially explain why visceral fat is a health risk.

Whitmer investigated the link between visceral fat and dementia. In a study, she evaluated the records of more than 6,500 members of Kaiser Permanente of Northern California, a large health maintenance organization, for an average of 36 years, from the time they were in their 40s until they were in their 70s.

The records included details on height, weight, and belly diameter—a reflection of the amount of visceral fat. Those with the biggest bellies had a higher risk of dementia than those with smaller bellies. The link was true even for people with excess belly fat but overall of normal weight.

She doesn't know why belly fat and dementia are linked, but speculates that substances such as leptin, a hormone released by the belly fat, may have some adverse effect on the brain. Leptin plays a role in appetite regulation but also in learning and memory.

## Belly Fat

Belly fat has gotten a mostly deserved reputation as an unhealthy fat. "Understand that belly fat is both visceral and subcutaneous," says Kristen Gill Hairston, MD, MPH, an assistant professor of medicine at Wake Forest University School of Medicine, Winston-Salem, N.C. "We don't have a perfect way yet to determine which [of belly fat] is subcutaneous or visceral, except by CT scan, but that's not cost-effective."

But if you've got an oversize belly, figuring out how much is visceral and how much is subcutaneous isn't as important as recognizing a big belly is unhealthy, she says. How big is too big? Women with a waist circumference more than 35 inches and men with a waist circumference more than 40 inches are at increased disease risk.

Abdominal fat is viewed as a bigger health risk than hip or thigh fat, Whitmer and other experts say. And that could mean having a worse effect on insulin resistance, boosting the risk of diabetes, and a worse effect on blood lipids, boosting heart and stroke risks.

## Thigh Fat, Buttocks Fat

While men tend to accumulate fat in the belly, it's no secret women, especially if "pear-shaped," accumulate it in their thighs and buttocks.

Unsightliness aside, emerging evidence suggests that pear-shaped women are protected from metabolic disease compared to big-bellied people, says Fried.

"Thigh fat and butt fat might be good," she says, referring to that area's stores of subcutaneous fat. But the benefit of women being pear shaped may stop at menopause, when women tend to deposit more fat in the abdomen.

## Weight Loss and Fat Loss

So when you lose weight, what kind or kinds of fat do you shed? "You're losing white fat," Fried tells WebMD. "People tend to lose evenly all over."

The results change a bit, however, if you add workouts to your calorie reduction, she says. "If you exercise plus diet you will tend to lose slightly more visceral fat from your belly."

"We're at an exciting point in science," says Whitmer, echoing the input from other scientists in the field.

Whitmer and others expect more discoveries about fat of all types to be made in the near future.

The basic idea we are proposing in this book is that maximizing melatonin will help to prevent obesity. This is not a new idea. This article from 1974 from the Max Planck Institute in Germany (one of the most renowned research centers of Europe) points out the evidence.[3]

---

[3] *Nature* 247 (January 25, 1974): 224–225, doi:10.1038/247224a0.

# Melatonin Stimulates Growth of Brown Adipose Tissue

Gerhard Heldmaier and Klaus Hoffmann

Max-Planck-Institut für Verhaltensphysiologie, D *8131* Erling-Andechs

IN small mammals brown adipose tissue (BAT) is an important site of non-shivering heat production[1] Its mass increases during cold adaptation together with the ability to produce heat ( G. H., unpublished), thus improving cold tolerance. In the golden hamster, Hoffman *et al.* also found an increase of BAT weight following exposure to short photoperiods. The pineal hormone melatonin has been shown to affect photoperiodic responses ( K. H. and G. H., unpublished), and therefore an action of melatonin on development of BAT seemed likely. In this study, the effect of short photoperiods and of melatonin on the amount of BAT was investigated in the Djungarian hamster *Phodopus sungorus*. This species shows a marked annual cycle of testis size and activity, body weight, and coat colour when kept under natural light conditions[7], and all of these functions can be influenced by manipulation of the photoperiod ( K. H. and G. H., unpublished). The species does not hibernate, but may show daily torpor in winter, while the gonads are regressed even at room temperature.

The following studies carried out thirty-nine years after the above study describe the details of how this works.

The following is a *Science News* article.

## Melatonin Helps Control Weight Gain as It Stimulates the Appearance of "Beige Fat" That Can Burn Calories instead of Storing Them, Study Suggests

*Sep. 25, 2013*—Spanish scientists have discovered that melatonin consumption helps control weight gain because it stimulates the appearance of "beige fat", a type of fat cell that burns calories *in vivo* instead of storing them. White adipose tissue stores calories leading to weight gain whereas "beige fat" (also known as "good or thinning fat") helps regulate body weight control, hence its metabolic benefits.

In the *Journal of Pineal Research*, scientists from the University of Granada Institute for Neuroscience, the Hospital Carlos III, Madrid, and the University of Texas Health Science Center in San Antonio (USA) have revealed, for the first time, the previously unknown enigma of why melatonin has metabolic benefits in treating diabetes and hyperlipidemia.

In earlier publications, the researchers analysed the effects of melatonin on obesity, dyslipidemia, high blood pressure and type 2 diabetes mellitus associated with obesity in young obese diabetic Zucker rats—an experimental model of metabolic syndrome.

In view of their most recent results, it seems the key lies in the fact that chronic melatonin consumption not only induces the appearance of "beige fat" in obese diabetic rats, but also increases its presence in thin animals used as a control group. "Beige fat" cells are found in scattered lentil-sized deposits beneath the inguinal skin in obese diabetic Zucker rats.

Melatonin is a natural hormone segregated by the human body itself and melatonin levels generally increase in the dark at night. It is also found in small quantities in fruit and vegetables like mustard, Goji berries, almonds, sunflower seeds, cardamom, fennel, coriander and cherries. These findings, together with the pharmacologically safe profile of melatonin, mean it is a potentially useful tool both in its own right and to complement the treatment of obesity. Sleeping in the dark and consuming these foodstuffs could help control weight gain and prevent cardiovascular diseases associated with obesity and dyslipidemia.

The study—coordinated by University of Granada lecturer Ahmad Agil—showed that chronic administration of melatonin sensitizes the thermogenic effect of exposure to cold, heightens the thermogenic effect of exercise and, therefore, constitutes excellent therapy against obesity. The fact is that one of the key differences between "beige fat", which appears when administering melatonin, and "white fat", is that "beige fat" cell mitochondria express levels of UCP1 protein, responsible for burning calories and generating heat.

The study—authored by Aroa Jiménez-Aranda, Gumersindo Fernández-Vázquez, Daniel Campos, Mohamed Tassi, Lourdes Velasco-Perez, Tx Tan, Russel J. Reiter and Ahmad Agil—has been part-financed and supported by the Granada Research of Excellence Initiative on BioHealth (GREIB), the University of Granada Vice-Rectorate for Scientific Policy and Research, and the regional government of Andalusia research group CTS-109.

Given the importance of this discovery, the researchers are confident they will obtain the funding needed to continue their work—says principle researcher Ahmad Agil—"and be able to achieve their final objective: to confirm these findings in humans, by administering melatonin to help combat obesity and diabetes.

The following *Science News* article describes where new brown fat might come from:

## Study Unlocks Origin of Brown Fat Cells, Important in Weight Maintenance

*Sep. 26, 2013*—In ongoing research aimed at battling obesity, UT Southwestern Medical Center researchers have deciphered how new fat cells are formed in energy-storing fat pads.

In particular, researchers sought to find out the origin of "brown" fat cells and whether humans can make more of them in order to burn extra calories—a finding that could have significant impact in battling obesity and related diseases.

"Much of the current excitement in the obesity field stems from recent observations highlighting that, even as adults, we have the ability to generate brown fat cells in response to cold exposure. Unlike white fat cells that mostly just store fat, brown adipocytes keep us warm by burning fat at a high rate," said Dr. Philipp Scherer, Director of the Touchstone Center for Diabetes Research at UT Southwestern and senior author of the study available online at *Nature Medicine*.

While generation of brown fat cells previously was thought to be mostly relevant for rodents and human infants, Dr. Scherer said, current evidence points to the observation that adults also generate these cells when exposed to cold.

Brown fat cells in adults tend to be randomly interspersed in subcutaneous white fat, with a trend toward increased accumulation in the upper chest and neck areas. In general, brown fat tissue makes up just a small percentage of total body fat mass.

The Touchstone Center's staff devotes its efforts to the study of cells and tissues that either contribute to, or are affected by, diabetes and its related diseases, including the physiology of fat tissue. In this study, the UT Southwestern research team examined the timing and nature of changes in fat cell composition in response to weight gain, cold exposure, and development. Genetic tools developed at the medical center over the past eight years were used to label all pre-existing fat cells. Researchers then were able to track where new fat cells emerged.

When mice were exposed to high-fat diets, significant differences between the types of white fat deposits were observed—subcutaneous fat deposits took their existing fat cells and made them bigger, while other deposits were more prone to generating new fat cells. Brown fat cells did not form during this experiment, nor during a test that monitored early growth-related development. Only when exposed to cold did new brown fat cells appear.

"The major finding is that the cold-induced adaptation and appearance of brown fat cells involves the generation of completely new cells rather than a retooling of pre-existing white fat cells into brown fat cells in response to the cold," Dr. Scherer said.

The researcher's next hope to translate these findings into clinical use, with future efforts directed toward therapeutic strategies to activate precursor cells to become new brown fat cells rather than to convert white fat cells into brown fat cells.

More information on brown fat stem cells is found in this *Science News* article.

## Newly Identified Brown Fat Stem Cells Hold Possibilities for Treating Diabetes, Obesity

*Nov. 21, 2013*—Obesity and diabetes have become a global epidemic leading to severe cardiovascular disease. Researchers at the University of Utah believe their recent identification of brown fat stem cells in adult humans may lead to new treatments for heart and endocrine disorders, according to a new study published in the peer-reviewed journal *Stem Cells*.

The study was led by Amit N. Patel, M.D. M.S., director of Clinical Regenerative Medicine and Tissue Engineering and associate professor in the Division of Cardiothoracic Surgery at the University of Utah School of Medicine.

Prior to Patel's study, it was thought that brown fat stem cells did not exist in adults. Children have large amounts of brown fat that is highly metabolically active, which allows them to eat large amounts of food and not gain weight. Patel notes, adults generally have an abundance of white fat in their bodies, which leads to weight gain and cardiovascular disease but this is not seen in brown fat. As people age the amount of white fat increases and brown fat decreases which contributes to diabetes and high cholesterol.

"If you have more brown fat, you weigh less, you're metabolically efficient, and you have fewer instances of diabetes and high cholesterol. The unique identification of human brown fat stem cells in the chest of patients aged from 28 to 84 years is profound. We were able to isolate the human stem cells, culture and grow them, and implant them into a pre-human model which has demonstrated positive effects on glucose levels," said Patel.

The new discovery of finding brown fat stem cells may help in identifying potential drugs that may increase the body's own ability to make brown fat or find novel ways to directly implant the brown fat stem cells into patients.

The current study will be presented November 22nd at the Annual Meeting of the International Federation for Adipose Therapeutics and Science (iFATS) in New York City. The study was sponsored in part by BioRestorative Therapies, Inc. (Jupiter, Florida.)

This *Medical News Today* article presents more evidence that it is the brown fat that helps get rid of excess calories.

## Lack of Brown Fat Linked to Diabetes Risk in South Asians

Tuesday 12 November 2013—12am PST

**Researchers have long known that people of South Asian origin have a higher risk of developing metabolic problems, such as type 2 diabetes. Now, a new study published in *The Lancet Diabetes and Endocrinology* suggests that lack of brown fat may explain why.**

According to researchers from the Netherlands, not only do individuals of a South Asian descent have an increased risk of type 2 diabetes and complications related to the condition, they also develop type 1 diabetes at a much younger age and at a much lower body mass index (BMI), compared with Caucasians.

However, it has previously been unclear as to why there are such differences.

The researchers looked to the effects of brown fat, also known as brown adipose tissue (BAT), for their study.

Monitoring the effects of brown fat

Pre-clinical studies have shown that brown fat has beneficial effects on glucose tolerance, lipid metabolism and body weight, and that brown fat activity is reduced in adults who are obese.

**Instead of storing the body's excess energy as fat—as white fat cells do—brown fat cells in brown adipose tissue convert some of this energy into heat when the body is cold. This burns excess energy as opposed to storing it.**

Previous research has estimated that fully functional brown adipose tissue accounts for up to 20% of a person's total energy usage.

The researchers analyzed 12 healthy South Asian men and 12 healthy Caucasian men of a normal weight who were approximately 25-years-old.

All of the men were exposed to cold temperatures using [18]F-fluorodeoxyglucose positron emission tomography and computed tomography ([18]F-FDG-PET-CT) scans.

The men's resting energy expenditure was monitored, alongside the effect of cold exposure on their non-shivering thermogenesis—increased heat production caused by normal metabolic processes—and plasma lipid levels.

Lower BAT and resting energy exposure in South Asians

**It was found that resting energy exposure in the South Asian participants was 32% lower, compared with the Caucasian participants, while the volume of metabolically active brown adipose tissue was 34% lower.**

The researchers also found that the South Asian participants had a higher shiver temperature upon cold exposure—at 10.9°C—compared with Caucasian participants—at 8.9°C, even though the South Asian participants had a higher total fat mass.

Furthermore, it was found that the South Asian participants had a lower cold-induced non-shivering thermogenesis, compared with Caucasian participants.

The study authors note that their findings show that producing more brown adipose tissue or increasing its activity could have "therapeutic potential" in South Asians.

**It could help them increase the clearance of glucose and fatty acids and help convert excess white fat into heat, they say, reducing their risk of diabetes.**

They add:

"We recently showed that BAT can be recruited in humans following 10 days of cold intervention. Future studies should be directed towards the efficacy of this strategy, as well as other options, such as medication, to increase BAT volume or activity.

These strategies might ultimately be useful for improving the metabolic phenotype in South Asians with type 2 diabetes or at high risk of developing the disease."

In a comment piece linked to the study, Michael Symonds, of the University of Nottingham in the UK, says that South Asians are now the "ideal target for therapeutical interventions that might offer proof-of-principle that enhanced BAT volume or function can have long-term health benefits against metabolic disease."

Medical News Today recently reported on a study detailing an implantable sensor that could monitor cancer and diabetes.

Written by Honor Whiteman

The following from a blog on the company's website describes how they are approaching obesity using brown fat stem cells.

**BioRestorative Therapies to Present Preclinical Data from Its ThermoStem(R) Brown Fat Stem Cell Program at Annual Meeting of the International Federation for Adipose Therapeutics and Science**

JUPITER, Fla.—(BUSINESS WIRE)—November 20, 2013

BioRestorative Therapies, Inc. ("BRT" or the "Company") (OTCBB:BRTX), a life sciences company focused on adult stem cell-based cellular therapies for various personal medical applications, announces that preclinical data on its ThermoStem(R) brown fat stem cell program will be presented November 22(nd) at the 11(th) Annual Meeting of the International Federation for Adipose Therapeutics and Science (iFATS) in New York City. The meeting will take place November 21–24 at the Conrad Hotel New York and will bring together leading scientists and decision-makers in the exciting field of adipose stem cell research to learn about the latest scientific, medical and technological advances.

BRT Chief Scientist and Vice President of Research and Development, Francisco Silva, will be presenting preclinical data from the Company's ThermoStem(R) program that focuses on treatments using brown fat stem cells for metabolic disorders and obesity, primarily for the prevention of type 2 diabetes.

"We are very excited to be presenting new data at such an important meeting. Acceptance of our research for presentation validates the scientific rigor of our approach to treating type 2 diabetes and other metabolic disorders, which have reached global epidemic proportions," said Mark Weinreb, CEO of BioRestorative Therapies. "BRT's presentation aligns with the meeting's emphasis on cutting-edge approaches and original data, focusing on science and technology that will expand our knowledge and future applications of adult adipose-derived stem cells around the world."

—ThermoStem(R) is a treatment using brown fat stem cells that is under development for metabolic disorders including diabetes and obesity. Initial preclinical research indicates that increased amounts of brown fat in the body may be responsible for additional caloric burning as well as reduced glucose and lipid levels.

# CHAPTER 3
## Cool Stuff

The following article suggests why using another trick to get the body to make more brown fat is worth thinking about.

**Could Warm Houses Be Making Us Fat?**

Katherine Martinko Living/Health

November 28, 2013

It's tempting to crank up the indoor heat during winter, but scientists say it could be making us fat. Keeping your house cool has benefits beyond reducing heating costs, because cold temperatures activate a substance called brown fat that adults carry on their upper back and neck. (Babies have it, too, since they can't shiver effectively.) Also known as brown adipose tissue, brown fat acts as an internal furnace that consumes many calories, unlike regular fat, which stores extra energy and calories. The only catch is that brown fat must be activated first in order to start burning calories, and cool temperatures can do that.

A new study from Britain links rising indoor temperatures to obesity. Central heating has become common in American and British homes since 1960, and room temperatures and obesity have risen simultaneously. The average temperature of living rooms in Britain was 64.9 degrees Fahrenheit in 1978, creeping upward to 70.3 degrees by 2008. Bedrooms in the U.K. were kept at 59 degrees in 1978 and climbed to 65.3 by 1996. U.S. bedrooms were 66.7 degrees in 1987, up to 68 by 2005.

The paper's lead author Fiona Johnson explains that people now heat their entire houses. Historically, only the main room with a woodstove or fireplace got really warm, while bedrooms stayed cool, but nowadays people don't have to adjust as they move through the house. Add the extra hours of commuting in a heated car, with less time spent outside, and suddenly our bodies lose their brown fat because it's never activated. Dr. Johnson explains: "It's kind of 'use it or lose it.' If you're not exposed to cold, you're going to lose your brown fat, and your ability to burn energy is affected. But you can get it back."

Former NASA scientist Ray Cronise has made similar discoveries: "We can use thermal temperature to super-charge weight loss...In environments as mild as 60 degrees, some of these people saw metabolism rates boost by as much as 20 percent." Tim Ferriss, author of *The 4-Hour Body*, explains how "thermal dieting"—taking cold showers, drinking ice water, going for frigid walks—can burn calories. Admittedly, it sounds a bit extreme, so I was relieved to see Dr. David Katz, a Yale professor, express skepticism, suggesting that if people are desperate to lose weight, it's best to focus on diet and exercise.

I grew up in a very cool house, where a wood-burning cookstove heated the main floor during the day and the bedrooms upstairs were frigid in winter. The rule was that, if I felt cold, I had to put on another layer of clothing before complaining. Usually that second sweater or pair of socks did the trick; I've realized that most people don't dress properly to handle a cool house, hence their thermostat addiction. I still like the idea of gradually turning down the heat, but mostly because it will save energy and money.

The following is a press release from the University of Texas Southwestern Medical Center.

## Study Unlocks Origin of Brown Fat Cells Important in Weight Maintenance

DALLAS—Sept. 26, 2013—In ongoing research aimed at battling obesity, UT Southwestern Medical Center researchers have deciphered how new fat cells are formed in energy-storing fat pads.

In particular, researchers sought to find out the origin of "brown" fat cells and whether humans can make more of them in order to burn extra calories—a finding that could have significant impact in battling obesity and related diseases.

"Much of the current excitement in the obesity field stems from recent observations highlighting that, even as adults, we have the ability to generate brown fat cells in response to cold exposure. Unlike white fat cells that mostly just store fat, brown adipocytes keep us warm by burning fat at a high rate," said Dr. Philipp Scherer, Director of the Touchstone Center for Diabetes Research at UT Southwestern and senior author of the study available online at *Nature Medicine*.

While generation of brown fat cells previously was thought to be mostly relevant for rodents and human infants, Dr. Scherer said, current evidence points to the observation that adults also generate these cells when exposed to cold.

Brown fat cells in adults tend to be randomly interspersed in subcutaneous white fat, with a trend toward increased accumulation in the upper chest and neck areas. In general, brown fat tissue makes up just a small percentage of total body fat mass.

The Touchstone Center's staff devotes its efforts to the study of cells and tissues that either contribute to, or are affected by, diabetes and its related diseases, including the physiology of fat tissue. In this study, the UT Southwestern research team examined the timing and nature of changes in fat cell composition in response to weight gain, cold exposure, and development. Genetic tools developed at the medical center over the past eight years were used to label all pre-existing fat cells. Researchers then were able to track where new fat cells emerged.

When mice were exposed to high-fat diets, significant differences between the types of white fat deposits were observed—subcutaneous fat deposits took their existing fat cells and made them bigger, while other deposits were more prone to generating new fat cells. Brown fat cells did not form during this experiment, nor during a test that monitored early growth-related development. Only when exposed to cold did new brown fat cells appear.

"The major finding is that the cold-induced adaptation and appearance of brown fat cells involves the generation of completely new cells rather than a retooling of pre-existing white fat cells into brown fat cells in response to the cold," Dr. Scherer said.

The researchers next hope to translate these findings into clinical use, with future efforts directed toward therapeutic strategies to activate precursor cells to become new brown fat cells rather than to convert white fat cells into brown fat cells.

The investigation received support from the National Institutes of Health and the American Diabetes Association.

Other UT Southwestern researchers involved in the study were lead author Dr. Qiong Wang, a postdoctoral researcher in internal medicine; Caroline Tao, a graduate student and student research assistant in internal medicine; and Dr. Rana Gupta, assistant professor of internal medicine.

Two companies have jumped on the brown fat bandwagon with products that exploit the new findings about cooled exercise. This is from the *Cool Fat Burner* blog.

The Cool Fat Burner BOOSTS **Adiponectin** Levels by 62%!!! **(Winter 2013)**

The drug companies are spending *millions* trying to figure out how to harness the power of the hormone **adiponectin**...without success.

In a recent experiment, the Cool Fat Burner (and Cool Gut Buster) were shown to **increase adiponectin by 62%**. This is HUGE news and a significant scientific breakthrough!!!

Adiponectin was discovered in 1995. Adiponectin is a hormone released by fat tissue. Why are drug companies trying to put adiponectin in pill form?

**Here's what adiponectin can potentially do: \*\***

* induce weight loss

* burn fat for fuel

* restore & increase skeletal muscle mitochondria

* increase insulin sensitivity

- reduce systemic inflammation

- fight heart disease

- fight certain types of cancer

- repair damaged DNA

- increase cellular longevity

An impressive list—imagine a pill that could do all that! (Be cautious of anyone claiming to sell a pill to increase adiponectin—at this time there is NO LEGITIMATE PILL OR SUPPLEMENT to increase adiponectin. Chances are, there won't be—it's difficult to synthesize, and is destroyed by digestion.) So how does one increase adiponectin? Exercise *usually* does…but not always (1, 2). A good night's sleep can help, at least some. Others claim Omega-3 fatty acids can help, but the science isn't clear. So what about a *significant and consistent* method to increase adiponectin…?

Recently, another groundbreaking experiment was done that showed that cold thermogenesis, via the Cool Fat Burner & Cool Gut Buster, can increase adiponectin by a whopping 62%!!!

## The Experiment:

No exercise or cold thermogenesis for 4–5 days leading up to the experiment.

Eat normally the night before. Eat absolutely no carbs or sugars the morning of.

Get the "before" blood drawn in the morning.

Return to hotel room, have the A/C cranked, put on the CFB/CGB, use at Moderate to Hardcore intensity for around 2 hours.

Get the "after" blood drawn.

## What *actually* happened:

"After returning to the hotel room, I was dismayed to find the A/C was barely working. It wasn't cold in the least. (Note in the video, you can see the A/C cover had fallen off!) It was too late to try and switch rooms; the "after" blood test was pre-scheduled. I also wanted to prove the CFB could work in only a few hours. And on top of all that, hotel 'checkout' was in 3–4 hours. So I had to make due [sic] with the room I was in and the time I had.

"I had 9 cold packs that barely fit in the small freezer in the mini-fridge in my room, but had 11 more packs I'd brought and had them stored in the front desk refrigerator the night before. Apparently, the front desk worker from the night before *had put all the packs in the refrigerator section, not the freezer—those packs were all half thawed!!!*

"This means I had less packs required for even a single set of CFB/CGB usage! (4 packs in the CFB, 6 packs in a 'Small'-sized Gut Buster—I had only 9 fully frozen packs from my room!) Coupled with the poor A/C, the odds were stacked against me. Would only one set of packs be enough, especially without air conditioning? If I drank some ice water, would that be enough?

"So due to the thermo-neutral room, and the lack of extra packs, my cold-stress session lasted only 1.5 hrs. I was still able to spend much of the time in 'Hardcore' intensity. The combination of Cool Fat Burner plus Cool Gut Buster, with some ice water, was enough. After the session I immediately drove back to the lab and had the 'after' blood work drawn, roughly 2hrs after the 'before' samples."

Adiponectin levels:

Before—**7.1 ug/ml** (time: 8:30am)

After—**11.5 ug/ml** (time: 10:50am)

That is an increase of 62% after only a few hours of using the Cool Fat Burner!

Another company providing equipment for cooled exercise is KewlFit Weight Management. The following is taken from their website: www.kewlfit.com (coolfitness?)

## Academic Research

Introducing a new way to burn calories faster and achieve enhanced athletic performance. Backed by research from many of the world's leading universities, the KewlFit brand of cooling vests was designed to help you achieve your fitness and weight loss goals.

Lose weight with the KewlFit Weight Management Vest that was designed after the Harvard Medical School study that used a 14°C Cooling Vest to stimulate Brown Adipose Tissue. This tissue has been found in most adults in the neck, spine and clavicle regions only after exposure to mild cold temperatures. Research shows that activated Brown Adipose Tissue through cool temperatures has the potential to burn several hundred calories a day.

Achieve better results from your training and workouts with the KewlFit Performance Enhancement Vest. This cooling vest was designed after medical research that shows cooling the body prior to, during and after athletic activity results in better endurance, bigger gains and the ability to have a greater heat storage capacity. Athletes in search of a legal athletic edge are now training with the KewlFit PEV.

## Cooling the Body for Weight Management

Brown adipose tissue is responsible for the successful defense of body temperature without shivering (American Journal of Physiology)

There is no doubt that active brown adipose tissue is present in adult humans (Obesity Journal)

Activation of thermogenesis is an anti-obesity tool that can be accomplished in a variety of ways including the recruitment and activation of brown adipose tissue. This method would be the more physiological and a more comfortable way in promoting thermogenesis (Stockholm University)

58°F (14°C) Cooling Vests reliably activate brown fat (Harvard Medical School)

Mild cold exposure can prevent increases in body weight (Obesity Journal)

Activated Brown Fat boosts the rate at which we burn calories by 20% (New England Journal of Medicine)

Activated Brown Fat may burn an extra 500 calories/day (Harvard Medical School) also quoted in interview

Three ounces of brown fat can burn several hundred calories/day (ObesityInAmerica.org)

A substantial loss of fat is induced by a combination of exposure to cold and exercise (American Physiological Society)

Dr. André Carpentier, an endocrinologist at the University of Sherbrooke in Quebec said, the brown fat burned about 250 calories over three hours when the subjects were chilled, but not to the point of shivering (University of Sherbrooke—Journal of Clinical Investigation)

Brown adipose tissue, depending on its thermogenic activity, may contribute to the control of body fat metabolism in humans (Obesity Journal)

Activated brown adipose tissue has the potential to contribute substantially to energy expenditure (New England Journal of Medicine)

Cold-exposure designed to minimize muscle-mediated shivering enhances brown adipose tissue oxidative metabolism as well as glucose and NEGA uptake in adult humans (The Journal of Clinical Investigation)

When the tissue is active, the uptake in brown adipose tissue is a main utilizer of glucose in the body, perhaps superceded only by the brain. If this correlates with metabolic activity, it is clear that active brown adipose tissue may play a significant role in the metabolism of at least a significant fraction of adult humans (American Journal of Physiology)

Brown adipose tissue was visible in the neck, supraclavicular region, chest and abdomen under PET-CT scanning only after the subject was exposed to mild cold exposure (New England Journal of Medicine)

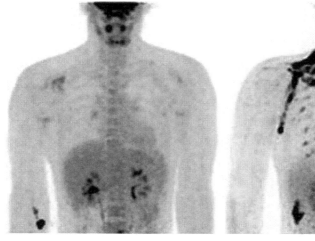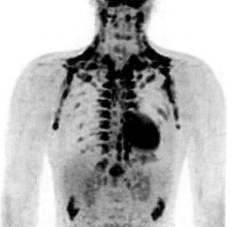

Brown Adipose Tissue active using PET-CT scan under cold exposure (right) and not active under non cold exposure (left)

# Cold Temperatures and Chili Peppers Help Burn Fat

By Douglas Main, Staff Writer, LiveScience Blog
October 17, 2013

What do low temperatures and chili peppers have in common? They both could help burn fat, a new study shows.

Exposure to cold and consumption of chemicals found in chili peppers both appear to increase the number and activity of so-called brown fat cells, which burn energy, rather than store it as typical "white" fat cells do, said Takeshi Yoneshiro, a researcher at Hokkaido University Graduate School of Medicine in Japan.

The study is the first to show that brown fat activity can be induced in people who appeared to have very few or no brown fat cells, said Dr. Clifford Rosen, a professor of medicine at Tufts University who wasn't involved in the study.

Participants in the study who were exposed to cold also had less "bad" white fat at the end of the experiments, Rosen told LiveScience.

## Cold burns fat

Brown fat cells are currently a subject of intense research as a target for anti-obesity drugs, said Dr. Soren Snitker, a medical researcher at the University of Maryland School of Medicine who wasn't involved in the study. [9 Myths That Can Make You Fat]

In the new study, researchers exposed eight people with little or no brown fat cells to moderately low temperatures of 63 degrees Fahrenheit (17 degrees Celsius) for two hours daily, over the course of six weeks. Compared with the control subjects, who went about their normal lives, the cold-exposed people had about 5 percent less body fat at the end of the study, and also burned more energy when exposed to cold, according to the study, which was published in August in the Journal of Clinical Investigation.

The researchers also looked at people who ate caps-inoids, which are normally found in chili peppers, for six weeks, and found they also burned more energy than the control group when exposed to cold, but didn't lose any more white fat than the control group.

Yoneshiro said the experiment might not have continued for long enough to see white-fat-burning effects of the compounds. A previous study that lasted 12 weeks found the capsinoid ingestion led to significant body fat decreases in mildly obese people.

The new results help explain the results from a recent study co-authored by Snitker, which found that people who ate capsinoids had increased levels of fat breakdown, and smaller waists after a six-week period, compared with people who took placebos.

## The brown and the beige

It was once thought that brown fat, also known as brown adipose tissue (BAT), was present only in babies. But three research groups independently discovered in 2009 that brown fat exists in adults, concentrated in the upper chest and neck of some adults, Rosen said. It appears reddish-brown because it contains many mitochondria, cellular factories that release energy, Rosen said.

In 2012, scientists found yet another type of BAT called "beige fat," which is a subset of brown fat but is formed from white fat cells. Rosen said that the "brown fat" cells induced by cold and capsinoids are indeed likely beige fat, because they don't show up on scans used to detect concentrated regions of brown fat cells.

"The most interesting thing about this study from a treatment point of view is the capsinoids," said Jan Nedergaard, a physiologist at Stockholm University in Sweden who wasn't involved in the study. Reduction of fat from cold exposure was expected, he said, but "as everybody realizes, that's a difficult thing to put into practice."

## Drug development?

The study is exciting because it suggests chemicals that induce brown fat could be used to fight obesity, although they'd probably work better at keeping healthy people from becoming fat, rather than making obese people skinny, Nedergaard said. "Everybody would like to take a fat person and make him slim, but that demands a high-burning capacity that BAT probably doesn't have."

Capsinoids appear to induce brown fat in the same way as cold, by "capturing" the same cellular system that the body's nervous system uses to increase heat production, Yoneshiro said. Drug developers want to use similar drugs to activate this system, but capsinoids themselves probably won't be used because they already exist in nature and thus cannot be patented, a major way that pharmaceutical companies make money, Nedergaard said.

Capsinoids come from "sweet" chili peppers that don't taste hot, but produce some of the same physiological effects—for example, producing sweat, Nedergaard said.

The stimulation of the metabolism from hot peppers is similar to that due to hyperthyroidism.

## Hyperthyroidism Increased Brown Fat Metabolism

Lahesmaa, M. J Clin Endocrinol Metab (2013), doi:10.1210/jc.2013-2312

November 1, 2013

Hyperthyroidism increased glucose uptake in brown adipose tissue independent of brown adipose tissue perfusion, according to follow-up study results published in the *Journal of Clinical Endocrinology and Metabolism.*

Researchers wrote that previous reports showed brown adipose tissue metabolism is upregulated by thyroid hormones in rats. Therefore, researchers carried out a study to measure glucose uptake and perfusion of brown adipose tissue, white adipose tissue, skeletal muscle and thyroid glands using PET imaging in 10 human patients with overt hyperthyroidism and eight healthy controls.

Patients with hyperthyroidism displayed a threefold greater amount of brown adipose tissue glucose uptake compared with healthy patients (2.7 mcmol/100 g/min vs. 0.9 mcmol/100 g/min; $P$=.0013), 90% higher skeletal muscle glucose uptake ($P$<.005), 45% higher energy expenditure ($P$<.005) and 70% higher lipid oxidation rate ($P$=.001), according to data.

However, the changes were reversible after restoration of euthyroidism, researchers wrote. During hyperthyroidism, serum free thyroxine and triiodothyronine were strongly associated with energy expenditure and lipid oxidation rates ($P$<.001). Thyroid-stimulating hormone had an inverse correlation with brown adipose tissue and skeletal muscle glucose metabolism ($P$<.001), according to data.

Hyperthyroidism had no effect on brown adipose tissue perfusion. However, it stimulated skeletal muscle perfusion ($P$=.04), researchers wrote. Thyroid gland glucose uptake did not differ between patients with hyperthyroidism and euthyroidism.

"These metabolic changes are similar to what is seen in response to insulin. During hyperthyroidism, activation of [brown adipose tissue] and skeletal muscle by thyroid hormones and simultaneous [sympathetic nervous system] activation may explain increased energy expenditure and higher use of lipids as energy substrate," researchers wrote.

Exercise also turns on brown fat.

## Exercise Can Turn "Bad" Fat into "Good" Brown Fat

Posted: 06/24/2013 3:37 pm EDT

Even if you aren't seeing results on your bathroom scale, exercise *is* making a difference in your health by turning "bad" fat into "good" fat, according to new research.

Studies presented at the annual meeting of the American Diabetes Association showed that both mice *and* men have beneficial "browning" of fat that comes from sedentary behavior if they exercise. For the mice, this came after 11 days of running on an exercise wheel; for the men, this came after 12 weeks of consistent exercise bike training.

Plus, when researchers tried transplanting the mouse's brown fat into other sedentary mice that had lots of fat, they found that the mice that received the fat transplant had improved insulin sensitivity and glucose tolerance. However, it remains to be seen if this benefit holds true for humans, too, since researchers are not yet able to transplant fat from one human to another in this way.

"Our results showed that exercise doesn't just have beneficial effects on muscle, it also affects fat," one of the researchers, Kristin Stanford, Ph.D., who is a postdoctoral fellow at Joslin Diabetes Center, said in a statement. "It's clear that when fat gets trained, it becomes browner and more metabolically active. We think there are factors being released into the bloodstream from the healthier fat that are working on other tissues."

Because both these studies have yet to be published in a peer-reviewed journal, they should be considered preliminary. But still, the Mayo Clinic points out that brown fat—which is "turned on" when a person gets cold—has gained the attention of researchers recently because it seems to burn calories.

In fact, a study published last year in the Journal of Clinical Investigation showed that cold temperatures seem to spur adult men's brown fat to burn calories; however, this calorie-burning effect didn't occur when the men were in warm temperatures.

## Melatonin Helps Control Weight Gain as It Stimulates the Appearance of "Beige Fat" That Can Burn Calories Instead of Storing Them, Study Suggests

*Sep. 25, 2013*—Spanish scientists have discovered that melatonin consumption helps control weight gain because it stimulates the appearance of "beige fat", a type of fat cell that burns calories *in vivo* instead of storing them. White adipose tissue stores calories leading to weight gain whereas "beige fat" (also known as "good or thinning fat") helps regulate body weight control, hence its metabolic benefits.

In the *Journal of Pineal Research*, scientists from the University of Granada Institute for Neuroscience, the Hospital Carlos III, Madrid, and the University of Texas Health Science Center in San Antonio (USA) have revealed, for the first time, the previously unknown enigma of why melatonin has metabolic benefits in treating diabetes and hyperlipidemia.

In earlier publications, the researchers analyzed the effects of melatonin on obesity, dyslipidemia, high blood pressure and type 2 diabetes mellitus associated with obesity in young obese diabetic Zucker rats—an experimental model of metabolic syndrome.

In view of their most recent results, it seems the key lies in the fact that chronic melatonin consumption not only induces the appearance of "beige fat" in obese diabetic rats, but also increases its presence in thin animals used as a control group. "Beige fat" cells are found in scattered lentil-sized deposits beneath the inguinal skin in obese diabetic Zucker rats.

Melatonin is a natural hormone segregated by the human body itself and melatonin levels generally increase in the dark at night. It is also found in small quantities in fruit and vegetables like mustard, Goji berries, almonds, sunflower seeds, cardamom, fennel, coriander and cherries. These findings, together with the pharmacologically safe profile of melatonin, mean it is a potentially useful tool both in its own right and to complement the treatment of obesity. Sleeping in the dark and consuming these foodstuffs could help control weight gain and prevent cardiovascular diseases associated with obesity and dyslipidemia.

The study—coordinated by University of Granada lecturer Ahmad Agil—showed that chronic administration of melatonin sensitizes the thermogenic effect of exposure to cold, heightens the thermogenic effect of exercise and, therefore, constitutes excellent therapy against obesity. The fact is that one of the key differences between "beige fat", which appears when administering melatonin, and "white fat", is that "beige fat" cell mitochondria express levels of UCP1 protein, responsible for burning calories and generating heat.

The study—authored by Aroa Jiménez-Aranda, Gumersindo Fernández-Vázquez, Daniel Campos, Mohamed Tassi, Lourdes Velasco-Perez, Tx Tan, Russel J. Reiter and Ahmad Agil—has been part-financed and supported by the Granada Research of Excellence Initiative on BioHealth (GREIB), the University of Granada Vice-Rectorate for Scientific Policy and Research, and the regional government of Andalusia research group CTS-109.

Given the importance of this discovery, the researchers are confident they will obtain the funding needed to continue their work—says principle researcher Ahmad Agil—"and be able to achieve their final objective: to confirm these findings in humans, by administering melatonin to help combat obesity and diabetes."

The following was taken from scienceblog.com/67924/fighting-obesity-new-hopes-from-**brown-fat/**

Richard L. Hansler, PhD

# Fighting Obesity: New Hopes from Brown Fat

November 19, 2013

**If you want to lose weight, then you actually want more fat, not less. But you need the right kind: brown fat. This special type of fatty tissue burns calories, puts out heat like a furnace, and helps to keep you trim. White fat, on the other hand, stores extra calories and makes you, well, fat. Wouldn't it be nice if we could instruct our bodies to make more brown fat, and less white fat? Well, NIH-funded researchers have just taken another step in that direction [1].**

A while ago, I told you about proteins that influence the development of brown fat cells, but the unraveling of this biological mystery continues. Today, I'm sharing the work of researchers at the University of California, San Francisco, who have discovered a key gene driving the engine of brown fat production. Even more exciting, they have linked mutations in this gene to obesity in humans.

A few years ago, members of this team discovered two master regulators of brown fat development [2]. When they inserted both of these genes into ordinary skin cells, they could reprogram the cells and transform them into brown fat. A major achievement, but neither of the genes

66

seemed to be a good target for drug therapy. So, they began to study one of the proteins, called PRDM16, in detail to figure out exactly how it coaxed precursor cells to become brown fat. In the newly published work, they found that PRDM16 needs to interact with an enzyme called EHMT1 to produce brown fat.

Searching a database of human genetic mutations, the researchers discovered that people with rare mutations in the EHMT1 gene are obese. That finding is important because it's the first evidence in humans suggesting that deleterious mutations in genes controlling brown fat production can cause obesity.

To probe EHMT1's activity, the UCSF team created a strain of mice in which the gene that codes for this enzyme was deleted, not from the whole animal, but just in the precursor cells destined to develop into brown fat. Without EHMT1, these precursor cells failed to develop into brown fat. The mice lacking EHMT1 were heavier than normal mice, even though they ate identical diets. They also had higher glucose levels, greater insulin resistance, and more fat in their livers—traits characteristic of diabetes and other metabolic diseases.

These findings suggest a new approach to treating obesity, which is urgently needed because more than one in three US adults are obese, and current treatments are far from ideal. Some anti-obesity medications suppress appetite, while others block fat absorption. But both types can cause undesirable side effects.

Moving forward, the UCSF group hopes to team up with collaborators to find chemical compounds that will activate the EHMT1 enzyme. If they succeed, perhaps we will someday be able to use medication to increase production of brown fat—and, in turn, burn up extra calories and white fat.

## References:

[1] EHMT1 controls brown adipose cell fate and thermogenesis through the PRDM16 complex. Ohno H, Shinoda K, Ohyama K, Sharp LZ, Kajimura S. *Nature*. 2013 Nov 6.
[2] Initiation of myoblast to brown fat switch by a PRDM16-C/EBP-beta transcriptional complex. Kajimura S, Seale P, Kubota K, Lunsford E, Frangioni JV, Gygi SP, Spiegelman BM. *Nature*. 2009 Aug 27;460(7259):1154-8.

The following article is from www.Nutraingreients.com

**Consumption of Melatonin Could Help Control Weight Gain by Stimulating the Development of "Beige Fat" Cells That Burn—Rather Than Store—Calories, Say Researchers**

The new study, published in the *Journal of Pineal Research*, noted that recent research has suggested that melatonin limits obesity in rodents without affecting food intake and activity—something that therefore indicates that the hormone may have a thermogenic effect.

Coupled with previous work that identified brown fat (or beige fat) in white adipose tissue (WAT) *"prompted us to investigate whether melatonin is a brown-fat inducer,"* explained the research team.

Led by senior author Ahmad Agil from the University of Granada, Spain, the team used a rat model to reveal that melatonin consumption is associated with the induction of beige fat that is known to help regulate body weight control, and offer metabolic benefits.

*"We report, for the first time, that oral melatonin supplementation induces browning of the inguinal WAT,"* the authors said.

Agil and his colleagues suggested that their results may also offer an insight in to the previously unsolved puzzle of why melatonin consumption has metabolic benefits for people with diabetes and hyperlipidaemia.

*"We have demonstrated that chronic melatonin treatment in rats behaves as a white fat browning inducer with thermogenic properties. This may be one of the mechanisms that underlies the antiobesity effect of melatonin and thereby explains its metabolic benefits, that is, antidiabetic and lipid-lowering properties,"* wrote the researchers.

## Research Study

*"Because melatonin treatment does not modify rat physical activity, it is presumed that it can potentiate the thermogenic effect of exercise,"* they said—adding that such an observation, coupled with the hormone's high pharmacological safety profile make melatonin *"a potentially useful tool for a stand-alone or adjunct therapy for obesity."*

## Study Details

The team used Zücker diabetic fatty (ZDF) rats—a model of obesity-related type 2 diabetes and a strain in which melatonin reduces obesity and improves their metabolic profiles.

At five weeks of age, ZDF rats and lean littermates (ZL) were subdivided into two groups, each composed of four rats: control and those supplemented with oral melatonin in the drinking water (10 mg/kg/day) for six weeks.

Melatonin supplementation was found to induce the browning of WAT in both ZDF and ZL rats.

The study also showed that chronic administration of melatonin sensitised the thermogenic effect of exposure to cold, and heightened the thermogenic effect of exercise. Therefore, the team suggested that melatonin supplementation may be an "excellent" therapy against obesity.

Given the importance of this discovery, Agil said that he is confident the team will obtain the funding needed to continue their work and be able to achieve their final objective: *"to confirm these findings in humans, by administering melatonin to help combat obesity and diabetes."*

Source: *Journal of Pineal Research*

Published online ahead of print, doi: 10.1111/jpi.12089

**Melatonin Induces Browning of Inguinal White Adipose Tissue in Zucker Diabetic Fatty Rats**

Authors: Aroa Jiménez-Aranda, Gumersindo Fernández-Vázquez, Daniel Campos, et al.

Melatonin May Offer Weight Management Potential: Animal Data

Consumption of melatonin could help control weight gain by stimulating the development of "beige fat" cells that burn—rather than store—calories, say researchers.[4]

The following is from *Women's Health*

**Melatonin for Weight Loss**
**Why Darkness Is Crucial for Weight-Loss**
**There may be a natural way to turn your bod into a calorie-burning machine, according to a new study.**

Published: October 3, 2013, by Elizabeth Narins

Why Darkness Is Crucial for Weight-Loss There may be a natural way to turn your bod into a calorie-burning machine, according to a new study

Want to lose weight? Turn off the lights. The sleep-promoting hormone melatonin can help your body produce a special kind of calorie-burning fat, according to an animal study recently published in *Journal of Pineal Research*.

---

[4] http://www.nutraingredients.com/Research/Melatonin-may-offer-weight-management-potential-Animal-data

In the study, a team of Spanish and American scientists fed 16 rats diets that were identical except for one difference: Some of the rats drank melatonin-enhanced water, while others drank regular water. At the end of the study, the researchers examined each animal's body for white and brown fat cells. (A primer: White fat stores calories and leads to weight gain, while brown fat burns way more calories than white fat and promotes weight loss.)

Interestingly, the rats that drank the melatonin-spiked water had more calorie-torching brown fat than white fat—even though their diets didn't change. Study co-author Russel Reiter, Ph.D., a professor at the University of Texas Department of Cellular and Structural Biology, says that melatonin can spark brown fat production and even turn some white fat into brown fat.

If these effects translate to humans (and Reiter says he thinks they would), melatonin could be the key to burning more calories without dieting. While previous research suggests that exercise and cold temperatures can trigger brown fat production as well, supplementing these efforts with melatonin is just plain easier—especially because you don't have to move more or freeze your butt off to see results. What's more: Melatonin is even safer than most OTC pain-killers, says Reiter. And while it's typically prescribed to promote sleep, it doesn't make people super-drowsy like other sleep aids.

Because there haven't been any human studies yet, though, it's unclear how much melatonin you'd need to take to see the number on the scale budge. The good news: Your body produces melatonin naturally in response to complete darkness. To boost your body's melatonin levels, just cut out all light at night: Invest in black-out bedroom shades, trash your nightlight, and keep the bathroom light (and your iPhone and iPad) off until the a.m. And if you're thinking of taking melatonin supplements to further boost your body's levels of the hormone, talk to a doctor first to make sure it won't have any adverse health effects.

In an effort to let people know about how using ordinary light at night was contributing to obesity, we (at John Carroll University and our partners in Photonic Developments LLC, the owners of www.lowbluelights.com) put out the following press release in 2012. There was very little evidence that anyone read it.

## Are Your Light Bulbs Making You Fat?

Obesity can result from chronic sleep deprivation and circadian disruption. Exposing the eyes to ordinary light in the hours before bedtime disrupts the circadian rhythm and prevents the flow of melatonin. Special light bulbs that block the blue rays that cause melatonin depletion are available at LowBlueLights.com.

University Heights, OH (PRWEB) July 30, 2012

There is a global epidemic of obesity with more than a billion people already overweight. It may seem ridiculous, at first, to suggest that ordinary light bulbs are to blame. However, many studies show a strong link between sleep deprivation, disruption of the circadian cycle and an increase in weight, especially in children (1). For example, obesity is much more common among night shift workers (2). But it is not just shift workers that are affected by exposure of the eyes to light at night. In our 24/7 lifestyle, we are all affected.

A very recent study (3) at the University of Surrey in the UK that was funded by Philips (the world's largest light bulb maker) found ordinary household lighting has a large negative impact on sleep. Studies at Harvard (4) found there is a large decrease in the amount of melatonin produced by exposure of the eyes to ordinary room light during the time the body would normally be producing melatonin. On average, people can produce melatonin for 11.5 hours a night if kept in darkness. Most Americans are in darkness for only 6 or 7 hours a night.

Fortunately, not all colors of light have the same effect on melatonin production. It is primarily the blue rays in ordinary white light that cause the problem. Light bulbs that don't produce the blue rays were developed by scientists at John Carroll University in 2005. Eyeglasses that block blue rays were also developed and are available at LowBlueLights.com. Thousands of people have purchased these products with a guarantee to get their money returned if the glasses do not improve their sleep. More than 90% of customers find the glasses or light bulbs improve their sleep.

Studies with animals have confirmed that exposure to too much light will cause them to get fat (5). The loss of melatonin due to light exposure (that causes the weight gain) can be avoided if melatonin is added to the animal's diet (6). Exactly how maximizing melatonin prevents obesity is not completely clear. One mechanism (7) involves the production of brown adipose tissue (fat). It can be converted to heat very readily in contrast to white fat. Melatonin stimulates both the production and conversion to heat of brown fat.

Undoubtedly obesity occurs when intake of calories exceeds their outgo. Maximizing melatonin to promote sleep and help convert fat to heat will be helpful. Avoiding blue light with special light bulbs or glasses in the hours before bedtime to maximize melatonin is an easy and inexpensive change in life style.

(1) de Jong E, Stocks T, Visscher TL, Hirasing RA, Seidell JC, Renders CM. "Association between sleep duration and overweight: the importance of parenting. Int J Obes (Lond). 2012 Jul 24. doi: 10.1038/ijo.2012.119. [Epub ahead of print]

(2) Association between sleep duration and overweight: the importance of parenting. de Jong E, Stocks T, Visscher TL, Hirasing RA, Seidell JC, Renders CM.

(3) Zhao I, Bogossian F, Turner C. (2)A cross-sectional analysis of the association between night-only or rotating shift work and overweight/obesity among female nurses and midwives. J Occup Environ Med. 2012 Jul; 54(7):834-40.

(4) Santhi N, Thorne HC, van der Veen DR, Johnsen S, Mills SL, Hommes V, Schlangen LJ, Archer SN, Dijk DJ. The spectral composition of evening light and individual differences in the suppression of melatonin and delay of sleep in humans. J Pineal Res. 2012 Aug;53(1):47-59. doi: 10.1111/j.1600-079X.2011.00970.x. Epub 2011 Oct 24.

(5) Gooley JJ, Chamberlain K, Smith KA, Khalsa SB, Rajaratnam SM, Van Reen E, Zeitzer JM, Czeisler CA, Lockley SW. Exposure to Room Light Before Bedtime Suppresses Melatonin Onset and Shortens Melatonin Duration in H (6)

(6) J Exp Pathol. 2007 Feb;88(1):19-29 Intake of melatonin is associated with ameliora-tion of physiological changes, both metabolic and morphological pathologies associated with obesity: an animal model. Hussein MR, Ahmed OG, Hassan AF, Ahmed MA.umans. (4) Clin Endocrinol Metab. 2011 Mar; 96(3):E463-72. Epub 2010 Dec 30.

(7) Wideman CH, Murphy HM. Constant light induces alterations in melatonin levels, food intake, feed effi-ciency, visceral adiposity, and circadian rhythms in rats. (5) Nutr Neurosci. 2009 Oct;12(5):233–40.

(8) Hussein MR, Ahmed OG, Hassan AF, Ahmed MA. Intake of melatonin is associated with amelioration of physiological changes, both metabolic and morpho-logical pathologies associated with obesity: an animal model. J Exp Pathol. 2007 Feb; 88(1):19–29.

(9) Ginter E, Simko V. Brown fat tissue—a potential target to combat obesity. Bratisl Lek Listy. 2012;113(1):52–6.

# CHAPTER 4
## The Plan: Putting It All Together

By now, you are probably thinking, *That's all very interesting, but how am I supposed to know what I need to do to avoid or treat obesity?* I hope it is now apparent to you that the place to start is in how you think about sleep. Sleep needs to become a very important part of your life, something you make plans to enjoy and treasure. Your bedroom needs to become the place where you sleep and enjoy sex and nothing more. It needs to be devoid of TV and off limits for electronic gadgets that provide both mental stimulation and exposure to blue light from their glowing screens. I don't recommend it, but if you still want to read in bed, use a low-blue-light lamp or book light. If you use an electronic device for reading, buy a blue-light filter for the screen.

The temperature in your bedroom should be cool but not so cold as to be highly uncomfortable. If it can't be a quiet place because of noise from traffic or neighbors, then it needs to be equipped with a source of white noise, such as that made by a fan or air conditioner. Lacking either of those, you can buy a commercial white-noise maker. While a clock may be necessary, it should not have a bright-blue numbers. If it does, buy a filter to block the blue rays.

Your bedroom should be dark. Opaque window shades are a must if you have streetlights or light from cars shining into your room. If you work shifts, you may need to have blackout-type blinds to get your bedroom dark enough to give you the benefit of sound sleep during the day.

Try to establish a regular, steady twenty-four-hour rhythm to your life. The constant disruption of the circadian rhythm is thought to be a major cause of obesity. Getting up at about the same time every morning and exposing your eyes to light at the same time every morning is the major way you can control your internal clock. This locks in your circadian rhythm. Developing a robust circadian rhythm in this way is key to good health.

Eating at the same times every day is also helpful. Your sense of hunger is very much under the control of the circadian clock. It is much easier to control how many calories you are putting into your body if you are eating on a regular schedule. If you can't resist snacking between meals, make it grapes, raisins, or nuts not chips or crackers.

The basic idea of this book is maximizing your production of melatonin by avoiding exposing your eyes to blue light for a number of hours before bedtime. In addition to making it easy to fall and stay asleep, it will also allow your body to produce brown fat and activate that fat to burn white fat to get rid of excess calories.

Turn down your thermostat. As you build up your supply of brown fat, you will be increasing your metabolism so you will be producing your own brown fat "furnace," which will allow you to be comfortable in a lower ambient temperature. Have you ever noticed young children running around in just a shirt and shorts and being warm as toast, while you're freezing even though bundled up in a wool sweater? Young children are still enjoying some of the brown fat they were born with. Helping our children to avoid blue light in the hours before their bedtime will, we hope, allow them to keep a good supply of brown fat and avoid obesity.

Exercise has also been shown to increase the amount of melatonin produced during the night. More melatonin means more brown fat. The exercise itself generates heat by burning fat so it has a double benefit. Some of the most recent studies suggest that exercising where it is cold will increase the amount of brown fat and thereby increase the benefit of exercise in terms of controlling weight. It is your call if you want to invest in cooling vests to wear while exercising. The theory sounds good, but I'm not ready to recommend their use just yet.

None of this allows one to ignore the basic facts that to lose weight, one has to have the calories "out" exceed the calories "in." Having brown fat available to help increase the calories "out" will be helpful but only if it is activated, so maximizing melatonin is vital, and staying in a cool environment will help. Reducing calories "in" is up to you. Living on a regular schedule will help you control what you eat.

I did promise to explain a couple of things. To start with, there is the business of how we know it's the blue rays that are the bad guys. Back in the eighties, Dr. George Brainerd was studying how light affects small animals. He knew that if the animals were kept under long night conditions, like fourteen hours of darkness and ten hours in the light, they were healthier than animals raised in the reverse, fourteen hours of light and ten hours of darkness. He wondered if the color of the light made any difference. He found that blue light was most effective in suppressing the production of melatonin in Syrian hamsters.

In 2001, he published the results of a similar study in humans that showed that the response curve was different for melatonin suppression than from that of either the rods or the cones. It peaked in the blue. A group at the University of Surrey was doing the same experiment and obtained identical results. They both had identified a previously unknown function for the eye. These newly discovered sensors did not provide vision but rather controlled the internal clock and the production of melatonin. It's surprising that it took until this new century to discover such a fundamental function of the eyes.

This business of keeping a regular rhythm of eating and sleeping and avoiding blue light is what, besides how much melatonin you make, seems to be important. It's referred to as circadian disruption. It's when your internal (or circadian) clock gets reset to a time different from the clock on the wall. This disruption of the circadian rhythm is thought by a number of scientists to be damaging to health, independent of loss of melatonin.

The balance of the book contains the scientific backup to what I have shared with you about how to develop a lifestyle that will help you to avoid or treat obesity. It is not light reading, but I hope you will have a look at what is there and read those abstracts that catch your interest. Free full papers are available for some of them. Putting the number at the end of the abstract in the search box at www.pubmed.gov will take you to the abstract and then to the free paper.

# CHAPTER 5
## Science behind how Melatonin Promotes Brown Fat

**Melatonin Induces Browning of Inguinal White Adipose Tissue in Zucker Diabetic Fatty Rats**

Jiménez-Aranda, A., G. Fernández-Vázquez, D. Campos, M. Tassi, L. Velasco-Perez, D. X. Tan, R. J. Reiter, A. Agil A. *J Pineal Res.* 55 no. 4 (November 2013): 416–23. doi: 10.1111/jpi.12089, Epub September 6, 2013.

## Source

Department of Pharmacology and Neurosciences Institute (CIBM), School of Medicine, University of Granada, Granada, Spain.

## Abstract

Melatonin limits obesity in rodents without affecting food intake and activity, suggesting a thermogenic effect.

Identification of brown fat (beige/brite) in white adipose tissue (WAT) prompted us to investigate whether melatonin is a brown-fat inducer. We used Zücker diabetic fatty (ZDF) rats, a model of obesity-related type 2 diabetes and a strain in which melatonin reduces obesity and improves their metabolic profiles. At 5 wk of age, ZDF rats and lean littermates (ZL) were subdivided into two groups, each composed of four rats: control and those treated with oral melatonin in the drinking water (10 mg/kg/day) for 6 wk. Melatonin induced browning of inguinal WAT in both ZDF and ZL rats. Hematoxylin-eosin staining showed patches of brown-like adipocytes in inguinal WAT in ZDF rats and also increased the amounts in ZL animals. Inguinal skin temperature was similar in untreated lean and obese rats. Melatonin increased inguinal temperature by $1.36 \pm 0.02°C$ in ZL and by $0.55 \pm 0.04°C$ in ZDF rats and sensitized the thermogenic effect of acute cold exposure in both groups. Melatonin increased the amounts of thermogenic proteins, uncoupling protein 1 (UCP1) (by ~2-fold, $P < 0.01$) and PGC-1α (by 25%, $P < 0.05$) in extracts from beige inguinal areas in ZL rats. Melatonin also induced measurable amounts of UCP1 and stimulated by ~2-fold the levels of PGC-1α in ZDF animals. Locomotor activity and circulating irisin levels were not affected by melatonin. These results demonstrate that chronic oral melatonin drives WAT into a brown-fat-like function in ZDF rats.

This may contribute to melatonin's control of body weight and its metabolic benefits.

PMID: 24007241

# Quantitative Proton MR Techniques for Measuring Fat

Hu H.H., and H. E. Kan. *NMR Biomed.* 26 no. 12 (December 2013):1609–29. doi: 10.1002/nbm.3025. Epub (October 3, 2013).

## Source

Department of Radiology, Children's Hospital Los Angeles, University of Southern California, Los Angeles, CA, USA.

## Abstract

Accurate, precise and reliable techniques for the quantification of body and organ fat distributions are important tools in physiology research. They are critically needed in studies of obesity and diseases involving excess fat accumulation. Proton MR methods address this need by providing an array of relaxometry-based (T1, T2 ) and chemical shift-based approaches. These techniques can generate informative visualizations of regional and whole-body fat distributions, yield measurements of fat volumes within specific body depots and quantify fat accumulation in abdominal organs and muscles. MR methods are commonly used to investigate the role of fat in nutrition and metabolism, to measure the efficacy of short- and long-term dietary and exercise interventions, to study the implications of fat in organ steatosis and muscular dystrophies and to elucidate pathophysiological mechanisms in the context of obesity and its comorbidities. The purpose of this review is to provide a summary of mainstream MR strategies for fat quantification. The article succinctly describes the principles that differentiate water and fat proton signals, summarizes the advantages and limitations of various techniques and offers a few illustrative examples. The article also highlights recent efforts in the MR of brown adipose tissue and concludes by briefly discussing some future research directions.

PMID: 24123229

## Dark Nights Reverse Metabolic Disruption Caused by Dim Light at Night

Fonken, L.K., Z. M. Weil, and R. J. Nelson. *Obesity* (Silver Spring) 21 no. 6 (June 2013):1159–64. doi: 10.1002/oby.20108. Epub May 10, 2013.

## Source

Department of Neuroscience and Institute for Behavioral Medicine Research, Wexner Medical Center, Ohio State University, Columbus, Ohio 43210, USA.

## Abstract

Objective:

The increasing prevalence of obesity and related metabolic disorders coincides with increasing exposure to light at night. Previous studies report that mice exposed to dim light at night (dLAN) develop symptoms of metabolic syndrome. This study investigated whether mice returned to dark nights after dLAN exposure recover metabolic function.

Design and Methods:

Male Swiss-Webster mice were assigned to either: standard light-dark (LD) conditions for 8 weeks (LD/LD), dLAN for 8 weeks (dLAN/dLAN), LD for 4 weeks followed by 4 weeks of dLAN (LD/dLAN), and dLAN for 4 weeks followed by 4 weeks of LD (dLAN/LD).

Results:

After 4 weeks in their respective lighting conditions both groups initially placed in dLAN increased body mass gain compared to LD mice. Half of the dLAN mice (dLAN/LD) were then transferred to LD and vice versa (LD/dLAN). Following the transfer dLAN/dLAN and LD/dLAN mice gained more weight than LD/LD and dLAN/LD mice. At the conclusion of the study dLAN/LD mice did not differ from LD/LD mice with respect to weight gain and had lower fat pad mass compared to dLAN/dLAN mice. Compared to all other groups dLAN/dLAN mice decreased glucose tolerance as indicated by an intraperitoneal glucose tolerance test at week 7, indicating that dLAN/LD mice recovered glucose metabolism. dLAN/dLAN mice also increased MAC1 mRNA expression in peripheral fat as compared to both LD/LD and dLAN/LD mice, suggesting peripheral inflammation is induced by dLAN, but not sustained after return to LD.

Conclusion:

These results suggest that re-exposure to dark nights ameliorates metabolic disruption caused by dLAN exposure.

PMID: 23666854

# Adipose Tissue Browning and Metabolic Health

Bartelt, A., and J. Heeren. *Nat Rev Endocrinol.* (October 22, 2013). doi: 10.1038/nrendo.2013.204. [Epub ahead of print]

## Source

Department of Genetics and Complex Diseases, Harvard School of Public Health, Boston, MA 02115, USA.

## Abstract

Accumulation of excess white adipose tissue (WAT) has deleterious consequences for metabolic health. The activation of brown adipose tissue (BAT), the primary organ for heat production, confers beneficial effects on adiposity, insulin resistance and hyperlipidaemia, at least in mice. As the amount of metabolically active BAT seems to be particularly low in patients with obesity or diabetes mellitus who require immediate therapy, new avenues are needed to increase the capacity for adaptive thermogenesis. In this light, we review the findings that BAT in human adults might consist of not only classic brown adipocytes but also inducible brown adipocytes (also called beige, brown-in-white, or brite adipocytes), which are phenotypically distinct from both white and brown adipocytes. Stimulating the development of beige adipocytes in WAT (so called "browning") might reduce adverse effects of WAT and could help to improve metabolic health. This article focuses on the development and regulatory control of beige adipocytes at the transcriptional and hormonal levels. Emerging insights into the metabolic role of beige adipocytes are also discussed, along with the developments that can be expected from these promising targets for therapy of metabolic disease in the future.

PMID: 24146030

## Differences in the Metabolic Status of Healthy Adults with and without Active Brown Adipose Tissue

Zhang, Q., H. Ye, Q. Miao, Z. Zhang, Y. Wang, X. Zhu, S. Zhang, C. Zuo, Z. Zhang, Z. Huang, R. Xue, M. Zeng, H. Huang, W. Jin, Q. Tang, Y. Guan, and Y. Li. *Wien Klin Wochenschr.* 125, no. 21–22 (November 2013):687–695. Epub October 22, 2013.

## Source

Division of Endocrinology and Metabolism, Department of Internal Medicine, Huashan Hospital, Fudan

University, 12 Wulumuqi Middle Road, 200040, Shanghai, China.

## Abstract

Background:

Previous studies have proven the existence of active brown adipose tissue (BAT) in adults; however, its effect on systematic metabolism remains unclear.

Aim:

The current study was designed to investigate the differences in the metabolic profiles of healthy adults with and without active BAT using positron emission tomography-computed tomography (PET-CT) scans in the un-stimulated state.

Methods:

A cross-sectional analysis was performed to assess the health of adults using PET-CT whole-body scans at Huashan Hospital Medical Centre between November 2009 and May 2010. A total of 62 healthy adults with active BAT were enrolled in the BAT-positive group.

For each positive subject, a same-gender individual who underwent PET-CT the same day and who had no detectable BAT was chosen as the negative control. Body composition was measured, and blood samples were collected for assays of metabolic profiles and other biomarkers.

Results:

In both the male and female groups, BAT-positive individuals were younger and had lower body mass indexes, fasting insulin, insulin resistance, and leptin, but a greater level of high-density lipoprotein cholesterol compared with the negative controls. In the male group, body fat content and levels of tumor necrosis factor-α were significantly lower in the BAT-positive than in the negative control group.

Conclusions:

The healthy adults with active BAT in an un-stimulated state had favorable metabolic profiles suggesting that active BAT may be a potential target for preventing and treating obesity and other metabolic disorders.

PMID: 24146327

# Significance and Application of Melatonin in the Regulation of Brown Adipose Tissue Metabolism: Relation to Human Obesity

Tan, D.X., L. C. Manchester, L. Fuentes-Broto, S. D. Paredes, and R. J. Reiter. *Obes Rev.* 12 no. 3 (March 2011):167–88. doi: 10.1111/j.1467-789X.2010.00756.x.

## Source

Department of Cellular and Structural Biology, the University of Texas Health Science Center at San Antonio, San Antonio, TX 78229, USA.

## Abstract

A worldwide increase in the incidence of obesity indicates the unsuccessful battle against this disorder. Obesity and the associated health problems urgently require effective strategies of treatment. The new discovery that a substantial amount of functional brown adipose tissue (BAT) is retained in adult humans provides a potential target for treatment of human obesity. BAT is active metabolically and disposes of extra energy via generation of heat through uncoupling oxidative phosphorylation in mitochondria. The physiology of BAT is readily regulated by melatonin, which not only increases recruitment of brown adipocytes but also elevates their metabolic activity in mammals. It is speculated that the hypertrophic effect and functional activation of BAT induced by melatonin may likely apply to the human. Thus, melatonin, a naturally occurring substance with no reported toxicity, may serve as a novel approach for treatment of obesity. Conversely, because of the availability of artificial light sources, excessive light exposure after darkness onset in modern societies should be considered a potential contributory factor to human obesity as light at night dramatically reduces endogenous melatonin production. In the current article, the potential associations of melatonin, BAT, obesity and the medical implications are discussed.

PMID: 20557470

This paper from 2003 shows that a melatonin antagonist stops the formation of brown fat in the Syrian hamster—indirect evidence that melatonin promotes the formation of brown fat.

**S22153, A Melatonin Antagonist, Dissociates Different Aspects of Photoperiodic Responses in Syrian Hamsters**

Pitrosky, B., P. Delagrange, M. C. Rettori, and P. Pévet. *Behav Brain Res.* 138 no. 2 (January 22, 2003):145–52.

## Source

Neurobiologie des Rythmes, UMR-CNRS 7518, Université Louis Pasteur, 12 rue de l'Université, 67000 Stras-
bourg, France.

## Abstract

In the Syrian hamster, short photoperiod (SP) induces
changes in several physiological functions (body mass,
reproduction, hibernation), and these responses involve
the pineal hormone melatonin. The present study investigated the effects of a melatonin antagonist, S22153, on
photoperiodic adaptation of male Syrian hamster. When
constantly released from subcutaneous implants, S22153
had no effect on body or testes masses of animals kept
in long photoperiod. S22153 decreased the total hibernation duration observed in animals exposed to SP and low
temperature. The decrease in hibernation duration was
due to a marked reduction in the number and duration of
hypothermic bouts. Moreover, S22153 significantly inhib-
ited the increase of interscapular brown adipose tissue
(BAT) mass induced by SP. However, neither the gonadal
atrophy nor the body mass increase induced by SP were
affected by S22153. These results show that S22153
affects only part of the physiological changes controlled

by SP and cold. Whether the decreases in BAT mass and hibernation duration are linked still remains an open question.

PMID: 12527445

## Significance and Application of Melatonin in the Regulation of Brown Adipose Tissue Metabolism: Relation to Human Obesity

Tan, D.X., L. C. Manchester, L. Fuentes-Broto, S. D. Paredes, R. J. Reiter. *Obes Rev.* 12 no. 3 (March 2011):167–88. doi: 10.1111/j.1467-789X.2010.00756.x.

## Source

Department of Cellular and Structural Biology, the University of Texas Health Science Center at San Antonio, San Antonio, TX 78229, USA.

## Abstract

A worldwide increase in the incidence of obesity indicates the unsuccessful battle against this disorder. Obesity and the associated health problems urgently require effective strategies of treatment. The new discovery that a substantial amount of functional brown adipose tissue (BAT) is retained in adult humans provides a potential target for treatment of human obesity. BAT is active metabolically and disposes of extra energy via generation of heat through uncoupling oxidative phosphorylation in mitochondria. The physiology of BAT is readily regulated by melatonin, which not only increases recruitment of brown adipocytes but also elevates their metabolic activity in mammals. It is speculated that the hypertrophic effect and functional activation of BAT induced by melatonin may likely apply to the human. Thus, melatonin, a naturally occurring substance with no reported toxicity, may serve as a novel approach for treatment of obesity. Conversely, because of the availability of artificial light sources, excessive light exposure after darkness onset in modern societies should be considered a potential contributory factor to human obesity as light at night dramatically reduces endogenous melatonin production. In the current article, the potential associations of melatonin, BAT, obesity and the medical implications are discussed.

PMID: 20557470


This paper is evidence that the lack of melatonin achieved by continuous light exposure results in production of excess body fat.

# Constant Light Induces Alterations in Melatonin Levels, Food Intake, Feed Efficiency, Visceral Adiposity, and Circadian Rhythms in Rats

Wideman, C.H., and H. M. Murphy. *Nutr Neurosci.* 12 no. 5 (October 2009):233–40. doi: 10.1179/147683009X423436.

## Source

Department of Biology, John Carroll University, 20700 North Park Blvd., Cleveland, OH 44118, USA.

## Abstract

Melatonin levels, metabolic parameters, circadian rhythm activity patterns, and behavior were observed in rats subjected to a 12-h/12-h light/dark cycle (LD) compared to animals exposed to continuous dark (DD) or continuous light (LL). LD and DD animals were similar in melatonin levels, food intake, relative food intake, feed efficiency, water intake, circadian activity levels, and behavior. LL animals had lower melatonin levels in the subjective dark compared to LD and DD animals. Food intake, relative food intake, and water intake values were lower and feed efficiency was more positive in LL animals compared to LD and DD animals. In addition, LL animals exhibited greater visceral adiposity than the other two groups.

The circadian rhythmicity of activity became free-running in LL animals and there was a decrease in overall activity. Notable behavioral changes in LL animals were an increase in irritability and excitability. Results indicate that a decrease in melatonin levels and concomitant changes in metabolism, circadian rhythms, and behavior are consequences of exposure to constant light.

PMID: 19761654

# CHAPTER 6
## The Science behind "Sleep Less, Get Fat"

Studies with mice reduce the time required to test a hypothesis. Sleeping less and exposure to light at night are essentially the same thing. When you are not sleeping, you are exposing your eyes to light.

## Dim Light at Night Disrupts Molecular Circadian Rhythms and Increases Body Weight

Fonken, L.K., T. G. Aubrecht, O. H. Meléndez-Fernández, Z. M. Weil, R. J. Nelson. *J Biol Rhythms* 28 no. 4 (August 2013):262–71. doi: 10.1177/0748730413493862.

## Source

Department of Neuroscience and Institute for Behavioral Medicine Research, Wexner Medical Center, The Ohio State University, Columbus, OH 43210, USA.

Richard L. Hansler, PhD

# Abstract

With the exception of high latitudes, life has evolved under bright days and dark nights. Most organisms have developed endogenously driven circadian rhythms that are synchronized to this daily light/dark cycle. In recent years, humans have shifted away from the naturally occurring solar light cycle in favor of artificial and sometimes irregular light schedules produced by electric lighting. Exposure to unnatural light cycles is increasingly associated with obesity and metabolic syndrome; however, the means by which environmental lighting alters metabolism are poorly understood. Thus, we exposed mice to dim light at night and investigated changes in the circadian system and metabolism. Here we report that exposure to ecologically relevant levels of dim (5 lux) light at night altered core circadian clock rhythms in the hypothalamus at both the gene and protein level. Circadian rhythms in clock expression persisted during light at night; however, the amplitude of Per1 and Per2 rhythms was attenuated in the hypothalamus. Circadian oscillations were also altered in peripheral tissues critical for metabolic regulation. Exposure to dimly illuminated, as compared to dark, nights decreased the rhythmic expression in all but one of the core circadian clock genes assessed in the liver. Additionally, mice exposed to dim light at night attenuated Rev-Erb expression in the liver and adipose tissue. Changes in the circadian clock were associated with temporal alterations in feeding behavior and increased weight gain. These results are significant because they provide evidence that mild changes in environmental lighting can alter circadian and metabolic function. Detailed analysis of temporal changes induced by nighttime light exposure may provide insight into the onset and progression of obesity and metabolic syndrome, as well as other disorders involving sleep and circadian rhythm disruption.

PMID: 23929553

## Dim Light at Night Exaggerates Weight Gain and Inflammation Associated with a High-Fat Diet in Male Mice

Fonken, L.K., R. A. Lieberman, Z. M. Weil, R. J. Nelson. *Endocrinology* 154 no. 10 (October 2013):3817–25. doi: 10.1210/en.2013-1121. Epub July 16, 2013.

## Source

Department of Neuroscience, Wexner Medical Center, The Ohio State University, 636 Biomedical Research Tower, 460 West 12th Avenue, Columbus, Ohio 43210.

## Abstract

Elevated nighttime light exposure is associated with symptoms of metabolic syndrome. In industrialized societies, high-fat diet (HFD) and exposure to light at night (LAN) often co-occur and may contribute to the increasing obesity epidemic. Thus, we hypothesized that dim LAN (dLAN) would provoke additional and sustained body mass gain in mice on a HFD. Male mice were housed in either a standard light/dark cycle or dLAN and fed either chow or HFD. Exposure to dLAN and HFD increase weight gain, reduce glucose tolerance, and alter insulin secretion as compared with light/dark cycle and chow, respectively. The effects of dLAN and HFD appear additive, because mice exposed to dLAN that were fed HFD display the greatest increases in body mass. Exposure to both dLAN and HFD also change the timing of food intake and increase TNFα and MAC1 gene expression in white adipose tissue after 4 experimental weeks. Changes in MAC1 gene expression occur more rapidly due to HFD as compared with dLAN; after 5 days of experimental conditions, mice fed HFD already increase MAC1 gene expression in white adipose tissue. HFD also elevates microglia activation in the arcuate nucleus of the hypothalamus and hypothalamic TNFα, IL-6, and Ikbkb gene expression. Microglia activation is increased by dLAN, but only among chow-fed mice and dLAN does not affect inflammatory gene expression. These results suggest that dLAN exaggerates weight gain and peripheral inflammation associated with HFD.

PMID: 23861373

The above results are for mice. Studies of humans show similar results. Metabolic syndrome is the combination of high blood pressure, high sugar level in the blood, and being overweight or obese.

## Short Sleep Duration as a Risk Factor for the Development of the Metabolic Syndrome in Adults

Chaput, J. P., J. McNeil, J. P. Després, C. Bouchard, A. Tremblay. *Prev Med.* 57 no. 6 (December 2013):872–7. doi: 10.1016/j.ypmed.2013.09.022. Epub October 5, 2013.

## Source

Healthy Active Living and Obesity Research Group, Children's Hospital of Eastern Ontario Research Institute, 401 Smyth Road, Ottawa, ON K1H 8L1, Canada. Electronic address: jpchaput@cheo.on.ca.

Richard L. Hansler, PhD

# Abstract

## Objective:

The objective of this study was to investigate the association between self-reported sleep duration and the incidence of features of the metabolic syndrome in adults.

## Methods:

A longitudinal analysis from the Quebec Family Study (Canada) was conducted on 293 participants, aged 18 to 65 years, followed for a mean of 6 years (until 2001). Participants were categorized as short ($\leq$6h), adequate (7–8h) or long ($\geq$9h) sleepers. The metabolic syndrome was defined according to the American Heart Association/National Heart, Lung, and Blood Institute's criteria. The hypertriglyceridemic waist phenotype was defined as high waist circumference ($\geq$90cm in men and $\geq$85cm in women) combined with high fasting triglyceride level ($\geq$2.0mmol/L in men and $\geq$1.5mmol/L in women).

## Results:

The incidence rates of metabolic syndrome and hypertriglyceridemic waist phenotype were 9.9% and 7.5%, respectively. Short sleepers were significantly more at risk of developing the metabolic syndrome (relative risk (RR): 1.74; 95% confidence interval (CI): 1.05–2.72) and the hypertriglyceridemic waist phenotype (RR: 1.82; 95% CI: 1.16-2.79), compared to those sleeping 7 to 8h per night after adjusting for covariates. However, long sleep duration was not associated with an increased risk of developing the metabolic syndrome or the hypertriglyceridemic waist phenotype (either unadjusted or adjusted models).

**Conclusion:**

Short sleep duration is associated with an increased risk of developing features of the metabolic syndrome in adults.

PMID: 24099879

Studies in which people were followed for a number of years (prospective) are probably more meaningful than "snapshot" studies.

**A Large Prospective Investigation of Sleep Duration, Weight Change, and Obesity in the NIH-AARP Diet and Health Study Cohort**

Xiao, Q., H. Arem, S. C. Moore, A. R. Hollenbeck, and C. E. Matthews. *Am J Epidemiol.* 178 no. 11 (December 1, 2013):1600–10. doi: 10.1093/aje/kwt180. Epub, September 18, 2013.

Richard L. Hansler, PhD

## Abstract

The relationship between sleep and obesity or weight gain in adults, particularly older populations, remains unclear. In a cohort of 83,377 US men and women aged 51–72 years, we prospectively investigated the association between self-reported sleep duration and weight change over an average of 7.5 years of follow-up (1995–2004). Participants were free of cancer, heart disease, and stroke at baseline and throughout the follow-up. We observed an inverse association between sleep duration per night and weight gain in both men (P for trend = 0.02) and women (P for trend < 0.001). Compared with 7–8 hours of sleep, shorter sleep (<5 hours or 5–6 hours) was associated with more weight gain (in kilograms; men: for <5 hours, β = 0.66, 95% confidence interval (CI): 0.19, 1.13, and for 5–6 hours, β = 0.12, 95% CI: -0.02, 0.26; women: for <5 hours, β = 0.43, 95% CI: 0.00, 0.86, and for 5–6 hours, β = 0.23, 95% CI: 0.08, 0.37). Among men and women who were not obese at baseline, participants who reported less than 5 hours of sleep per night had an approximately 40% higher risk of developing obesity than did those who reported 7–8 hours of sleep (for men, odds ratio = 1.45, 95% CI: 1.06, 1.99; for women, odds ratio = 1.37, 95% CI: 1.04, 1.79). The association between short sleep and excess weight gain was generally consistent across different categories of age, educational level, smoking status, baseline body mass index, and physical activity level.

PMID: 24049160

## Seven to Eight Hours of Sleep a Night Is Associated with a Lower Prevalence of the Metabolic Syndrome and Reduced Overall Cardiometabolic Risk in Adults

Chaput, J. P., J. McNeil, J. P. Després, C. Bouchard, and A. Tremblay. *PLoS One.* 8 no. 9 (September 5, 2013): e72832. doi: 10.1371/journal.pone.0072832.

## Source

Healthy Active Living and Obesity Research Group, Children's Hospital of Eastern Ontario Research Institute, Ottawa, Ontario, Canada.

## Abstract

### Background:

Previous studies looking at the relationship between sleep duration and the metabolic syndrome have only used a dichotomous approach (presence/absence) and failed to adjust for important confounding factors.

The objective of the present study was to examine the association between self-reported sleep duration and features of the metabolic syndrome in adults.

**Methods:**

A cross-sectional analysis from the Quebec Family Study (Canada) was conducted on 810 participants aged 18 to 65 years. Participants were categorized as short (≤6 h), adequate (7–8 h) or long (≥9 h) sleepers. The metabolic syndrome was defined according to the American Heart Association/ National Heart, Lung, and Blood Institute's criteria.

**Results:**

Overall, 24.6% of the sample had the metabolic syndrome. A U-shaped relationship between sleep duration and the prevalence of metabolic syndrome (33.3%, 22.0% and 28.8% in short, adequate and long sleepers, respectively) was observed ($P<0.01$). Only short sleepers had a significant increase in the odds of having the metabolic syndrome (OR=1.76, 95% CI=1.08–2.84) compared to adequate sleepers after adjustment for age, sex, smoking habits, highest education level, total annual family income, alcohol consumption, coffee intake, menopausal status, daily caloric intake, and moderate-to-vigorous physical activity. Likewise, the clustered cardiometabolic risk score (i.e. continuous risk score based on the metabolic syndrome components) was significantly higher in short sleepers compared to adequate sleepers after adjustment for covariates (P<0.05).

## Conclusion:

Sleeping ≤6 h per night is associated with an elevated cardiometabolic risk score and an increase in the odds of having the metabolic syndrome after adjusting for possible confounders. These results strongly suggest that short sleep duration is a risk factor for the metabolic syndrome.

PMID: 24039808

## Short Sleep Duration Is Independently Associated with Overweight and Obesity in Quebec Children

Chaput, J.P., M. Lambert, K. Gray-Donald, J. J. McGrath, M. S. Tremblay, J. O'Loughlin, and A. Tremblay. *Can J Public Health.* 102 no. 5 (September-October 2011): 369–74.

## Source

Children's Hospital of Eastern Ontario Research Institute, Ottawa, ON.

## Abstract

### Objective:

To investigate the association of sleep duration with adiposity and to determine if caloric intake and physical activity mediate this relationship.

### Methods:

The Quebec Adiposity and Lifestyle Investigation in Youth (QUALITY) study is an ongoing longitudinal investigation of Caucasian children with at least one obese biological parent. Children (n = 550) with an average age of 9.6 years (SD = 0.9) who provided complete data at baseline were included in the cross-sectional analyses. Objective measures of adiposity (BMI Z-score, waist circumference, percent body fat measured by dual-energy X-ray absorptiometry), sleep duration and physical activity (accelerometer over 7 days), and diet (24-hour food recalls) were collected. Children were categorized into 4 groups according to sleep duration: < 10 hours, 10–10.9 hours, 11–11.9 hours, and > or = 12 hours of sleep per night.

### Results:

We observed a U-shaped relationship between sleep duration and all adiposity indices. None of energy

114

intake, snacking, screen time or physical activity intensity differed significantly between sleep categories. After adjusting for age, sex, Tanner stage, highest educational level of the parents, total annual family income, and parental BMI, only short-duration sleepers (< 10 hours) had an increased odds of overweight/obesity (OR 2.08, 95% CI 1.16–3.67). Addition of total energy intake and physical activity to the model did not change the association substantially (OR 2.05, 95% CI 1.15–3.63).

**Conclusion:**

The present study provides evidence that short sleep duration is a risk factor for overweight and obesity in children, independent of potential covariates. These results further emphasize the need to add sleep duration to the determinants of obesity.

PMID: 22032104

**The Association between Short Sleep Duration and Weight Gain Is Dependent on Disinhibited Eating Behavior in Adults**

Chaput, J.P., J. P. Després, C. Bouchard, and A. Tremblay. *Sleep*. 34 no. 10 (October 1, 2011):1291–7. doi: 10.5665/SLEEP.1264.

## Source

Children's Hospital of Eastern Ontario Research Institute, Ottawa, ON, Canada.

## Abstract

### Study Objective:

To investigate whether the relationship between short sleep duration and subsequent body weight gain is influenced by disinhibited eating behavior.

### Design:

Six-year longitudinal study.

### Setting:

Community setting.

### Participants:

Two hundred seventy-six adults aged 21 to 64 years from the Quebec Family Study.

## Measurements and Results:

Body composition measurements, self-reported sleep duration, and disinhibition eating behavior trait (Three-Factor Eating Questionnaire) were determined at both baseline and after 6 years. For each sleep-duration group (short- [≤6 h] average, [7–8 h], and long- [≥9 h] duration sleepers), differences in weight gain and waist circumference were tested by comparing the lowest (score ≤ 3) versus the highest (score ≥ 6) disinhibition eating behavior tertiles using analysis of covariance, with adjustment for potential confounding factors. Individuals having both short sleep duration and high disinhibition eating behavior were more likely to gain weight and increase their abdominal circumference over time ($P<0.05$); however, short-duration sleepers having a low disinhibition eating behavior trait were not more likely to increase their adiposity indicators than were average-duration sleepers. Over the 6-year follow-up period, the incidence of overweight/obesity for short-duration sleepers with a high disinhibition eating behavior trait was 2.5 times more frequent than for short-duration sleepers with a low disinhibition eating behavior trait. Energy intake was significantly higher in short-duration sleepers with a high disinhibition eating behavior trait ($P<0.05$ versus all other groups).

**Conclusions:**

We observed that having a high disinhibition eating behavior trait significantly increased the risk of overeating and gaining weight in adults characterized by short sleep duration. This observation is novel and might explain the interindividual differences in weight gain associated with short sleep duration.

PMID: 21966060

## Short Sleep Duration as a Possible Cause of Obesity: Critical Analysis of the Epidemiological Evidence

Nielsen, L.S., K. V. Danielsen, T. I. Sørensen. *Obes Rev.* 12 no. 2 (February 2011):78–92. doi: 10.1111/j.1467-789X.2010.00724.x.

## Source

Institute of Preventive Medicine, Copenhagen University Hospitals, Copenhagen, Denmark.

## Abstract

Systematic literature search for epidemiological evidence for an association of short sleep with weight gain and eventual development of obesity provided 71 original studies and seven reviews of various subsets of these studies. We have summarized the evidence for such an association with particular emphasis on prospective studies. The studies showed that short sleep duration is consistently associated with development of obesity in children and young adults, but not consistently so in older adults. We have identified critical aspects of the evidence, and assessed the possibility for interpretation of the evidence in terms of causality. We have discussed the requirement of temporal sequence between putative exposure and outcome and the implications of the time lag between them, the problems in adequate measurements of exposure and effects, the possible bidirectional causal effects, the necessary distinction between confounders and mediators, the possible confounding by weight history, and the possibility of common or upstream underlying causes. In conclusion, causal interpretation of the association is hampered by fundamental conceptual and methodological problems. Experimental studies may elucidate mechanisms, but adequate coverage of the entire pathway from sleep curtailment through obesity development is not feasible. Randomized trials are needed to assess the value of targeted interventions.

PMID: 20345429

# CHAPTER 7
# The Science behind How Exercise Helps Control Weight

**Exercise Attenuates the Metabolic Effects of Dim Light at Night**

Fonken, L.K., O. H. Meléndez-Fernández, Z. M. Weil, and R. J. Nelson RJ. *Physiol Behav.* 124C (October 30, 2013):33–36. doi: 10.1016/j.physbeh.2013.10.022. [Epub ahead of print]

## Source

Department of Neuroscience, Wexner Medical Center, The Ohio State University, Columbus, OH 43210, USA; Institute for Behavioral Medicine Research, Wexner Medical Center, The Ohio State University, Columbus, OH 43210, USA. Electronic address: fonken.1@osu.edu.

## Abstract

Most organisms display circadian rhythms that coordinate complex physiological and behavioral processes to optimize energy acquisition, storage, and expenditure. Disruptions to the circadian system with environmental manipulations such as nighttime light exposure alter metabolic energy homeostasis. Exercise is known to strengthen circadian rhythms and to prevent weight gain. Therefore, we hypothesized providing mice a running wheel for voluntary exercise would buffer against the effects of light at night (LAN) on weight gain. Mice were maintained in either dark (LD) or dim (dLAN) nights and provided either a running wheel or a locked wheel. Mice exposed to dim, rather than dark, nights increased weight gain. Access to a functional running wheel prevented body mass gain in mice exposed to dLAN. Voluntary exercise appeared to limit weight gain independently of rescuing changes to the circadian system caused by dLAN; increases in daytime food intake induced by dLAN were not diminished by increased voluntary exercise. Furthermore, although all of the LD mice displayed a 24h rhythm in wheel running, nearly half (4 out of 9) of the dLAN mice did not display a dominant 24h rhythm in wheel running. These results indicate that voluntary exercise can prevent weight gain induced by dLAN without rescuing circadian rhythm disruptions.

PMID: 24184414

N Engl J Med. 2009 Apr 9;360(15):1500-8. doi: 10.1056/NEJMoa0808718.

# Cold-activated brown adipose tissue in healthy men.

van Marken Lichtenbelt WD, Vanhommerig JW, Smulders NM, Drossaerts JM, Kemerink GJ, Bouvy ND, Schrauwen P, Teule GJ.

## Background

Studies in animals indicate that brown adipose tissue is important in the regulation of body weight, and it is possible that individual variation in adaptive thermogenesis can be attributed to variations in the amount or activity of brown adipose tissue.

Until recently, the presence of brown adipose tissue was thought to be relevant only in small mammals and infants, with negligible physiologic relevance in adult humans.

We performed a systematic examination of the presence, distribution, and activity of brown adipose tissue in lean and obese men during exposure to cold temperature.

Brown-adipose-tissue activity was studied in relation to body composition and energy metabolism.

## Methods

We studied 24 healthy men—10 who were lean (body-mass index [BMI] [the weight in kilograms divided by the square of the height in meters], <25) and 14 who were overweight or obese (BMI, ≥25)—under thermoneutral conditions (22°C) and during mild cold exposure (16°C). Putative brown-adipose-tissue activity was determined with the use of integrated 18F-fluorodeoxyglucose positron-emission tomography and computed tomography. Body composition and energy expenditure were measured with the use of dual-energy x-ray absorptiometry and indirect calorimetry.

## Results

Brown-adipose-tissue activity was observed in 23 of the 24 subjects (96%) during cold exposure but not under thermoneutral conditions. The activity was significantly lower in the overweight or obese subjects than in the lean subjects (P = 0.007). BMI and percentage of body fat both had significant negative correlations with brown adipose tissue, whereas resting metabolic rate had a significant positive correlation.

## Conclusions

The percentage of young men with brown adipose tissue is high, but its activity is reduced in men who are overweight or obese. Brown adipose tissue may be metabolically important in men, and the fact that it is reduced yet present in most overweight or obese subjects may make it a target for the treatment of obesity.

## The Effects of Acute and Chronic Exercise on PGC-1α, Irisin and Browning of Subcutaneous Adipose Tissue in Humans.

Norheim, F., T. M. Langleite, M. Hjorth, T. Holen, A. Kielland, H. K. Stadheim, H. L. Gulseth, K. I. Birkeland, J. Jensen, C. A. Drevon. *FEBS J.* November 15, 2013. doi: 10.1111/febs.12619. [Epub ahead of print]

## Source

Department of Nutrition, Institute of Basic Medical Sciences, Faculty of Medicine, University of Oslo, Oslo, Norway.

## Abstract

Irisin was first identified as a peroxisome proliferator-activated receptor γ co-activator-1 α (PGC-1α)-dependent myokine with the potential to induce murine brown-fat-like development of white adipose tissue. In humans, the regulatory effect of training on muscle FNDC5 mRNA expression and subsequently irisin levels in plasma is more controversial. We recruited

26 inactive men (13 normoglycaemic and normal weight = controls, and 13 slightly hyperglycaemic and over-weight = prediabetes group) aged 40-65 y for a 12 w intervention of combined endurance- and strength-training with 4 sessions of training/week. Before and after the 12 w intervention period, participants were exposed to an acute endurance work-load of 45 min at 70% of $VO_2$ max, and muscle biopsies were taken prior to and after exercise. Skeletal muscles mRNA for PGC1A and FNDC5 correlated and both PGC1A and FNDC5 mRNA levels increased after 12 w of training in both control and prediabetes subjects. Circulating irisin was reduced in response to 12 w of training, and was increased acutely (~1.2-fold) just after acute exercise. Plasma concentration of irisin was higher in prediabetes subjects compared to controls. There were little effects of 12 w of training on selected browning genes in subcu-taneous adipose tissue. UCP1 mRNA did not correlate with FNDC5 expression in subcutaneous adipose tissue or skeletal muscle or with irisin levels in plasma. We observed no enhancing effect of long-term training on circulating irisin levels, and little or no effect of training on browning of subcutaneous white adipose tissue in humans.

PMID: 24237962

## Exercise and Melatonin in Humans: Reciprocal Benefits

Escames, G., G. Ozturk, B. Baño-Otálora, M. J. Pozo, J. A. Madrid, R. J. Reiter, E. Serrano, M. Concepción, and D. Acuña-Castroviejo. *J Pineal Res.* 52 no. 1 (January 2012):1–11. doi: 10.1111/j.1600-079X.2011.00924.x. Epub August 16, 2011.

## Source

Centro de Investigación Biomédica, Parque Tecnológico de Ciencias de la Salud, Universidad de Granada, Granada, Spain.

## Abstract

The aim of this review is to update the reader as to the association between physical exercise and melatonin, and to clarify how the melatonin rhythm may be affected by different types of exercise. Exercise may act as a zeitgeber, although the effects of exercise on the human circadian system are only now being explored. Depending on the time of the day, on the intensity of light, and on the proximity of the exercise to the onset or decline of the circadian production of melatonin, the consequence of exercise on the melatonin rhythm varies. Moreover, especially strenuous exercise per se induces an increased oxidative stress that in turn may affect melatonin levels in the peripheral circulation because indole is rapidly used to combat free radical damage. On the other hand, melatonin also may influence physical performance, and thus, there are mutually interactions between exercise and melatonin production which may be beneficial.

PMID: 21848991

**Fatness Leads to Inactivity, but Inactivity Does Not Lead to Fatness: A Longitudinal Study in Children (Earlybird 45)**

Metcalf, B.S., J. Hosking, A. N. Jeffery, L. D. Voss, W. Henley, and T. J. Wilkin. *Arch Dis Child.* 96 no. 10 (October 2011):942–7. doi: 10.1136/adc.2009.175927. Epub June 23, 2010.

## Source

Department of Endocrinology and Metabolism, Peninsula Medical School, University Medicine, Level 7, Derriford Hospital, Plymouth PL6 8DH, UK.

## Abstract

Objective:

To establish in children whether inactivity is the cause of fatness or fatness the cause of inactivity.

Design:

A non-intervention prospective cohort study examining children annually from 7 to 10 years. Baseline versus change to follow-up associations were used to examine the direction of causality.

Setting:

Plymouth, England.

Participants:

202 children (53% boys, 25% overweight/obese) recruited from 40 Plymouth primary schools as part of the Early-Bird study.

Main Outcome Measures:

Physical activity (PA) was measured using Actigraph accelerometers. The children wore the accelerometers for 7 consecutive days at each annual time point. Two components of PA were analysed: the total volume of PA and the time spent at moderate and vigorous intensities. Body fat per cent (BF%) was measured annually by dual energy x ray absorptiometry.

Results:

BF% was predictive of changes in PA over the following 3 years, but PA levels were not predictive of subsequent changes in BF% over the same follow-up period. Accordingly, a 10% higher BF% at age 7 years predicted a relative decrease in daily moderate and vigorous intensities of 4 min from age 7 to 10 years ($r=-0.17$, $p=0.02$), yet more PA at 7 years did not predict a relative decrease in BF% between 7 and 10 years ($r=-0.01$, $p=0.8$).

Conclusions:

Physical inactivity appears to be the result of fatness rather than its cause. This reverse causality may explain why attempts to tackle childhood obesity by promoting PA have been largely unsuccessful.

PMID: 20573741

## Physical Activity Intensity, Sedentary Time, and Body Composition in Preschoolers

Collings, P.J., S. Brage, C. L. Ridgway, N. C. Harvey, K. M. Godfrey, H. M. Inskip, C. Cooper, N. J. Wareham, and U. Ekelund. *Am J Clin Nutr.* 97 no. 5 (May 2013):1020–8. doi: 10.3945/ajcn.112.045088. Epub April 3, 2013.

## Source

Medical Research Council Epidemiology Unit, Institute of Metabolic Science, Cambridge, United Kingdom.

## Abstract

Background:

Detailed associations between physical activity (PA) sub-components, sedentary time, and body composition in preschoolers remain unclear.

Objective:

We examined the magnitude of associations between objectively measured PA subcomponents and sedentary time with body composition in 4-y-old children.

Design:

We conducted a cross-sectional study in 398 preschool children recruited from the Southampton Women's Survey. PA was measured by using accelerometry, and body composition was measured by using dual-energy X-ray absorptiometry. Associations between light physical activity, moderate physical activity (MPA), vigorous physical activity (VPA), and moderate-to-vigorous physical activity (MVPA) intensity; sedentary time; and body composition were analyzed by using repeated-measures linear regression with adjustment for age, sex, birth weight, maternal education, maternal BMI, smoking during pregnancy, and sleep duration. Sedentary time and PA were also mutually adjusted for one another to determine whether they were independently related to adiposity.

Results:

VPA was the only intensity of PA to exhibit strong inverse associations with both total adiposity [P < 0.001 for percentage of body fat and fat mass index (FMI)] and abdominal adiposity (P = 0.002 for trunk FMI). MVPA was inversely associated with total adiposity (P = 0.018 for percentage of body fat; P = 0.022 for FMI) but only because of the contribution of VPA, because MPA was unrelated to fatness (P ≥ 0.077). No associations were shown between the time spent sedentary and body composition (P ≥ 0.11).

Conclusions:

In preschoolers, the time spent in VPA is strongly and independently associated with lower adiposity. In contrast, the time spent sedentary and in low-to-moderate-intensity PA was unrelated to adiposity. These results indicate that efforts to challenge pediatric obesity may benefit from prioritizing VPA.

PMID: 23553158

# CHAPTER 8
## The Science behind the Beneficial Effects of Cold

**Cold Acclimation Recruits Human Brown Fat and Increases Nonshivering Thermogenesis**

Van der Lans, A. A., J. Hoeks, B. Brans, G. H. Vijgen, M. G. Visser, M. J. Vosselman, J. Hansen, J. A. Jörgensen, J. Wu, F. M. Mottaghy, P. Schrauwen, and W. D. van Marken Lichtenbelt. *J Clin Invest.* 123 no. 8 (August 1, 2013):3395–403. doi: 10.1172/JCI68993. Epub July 15, 2013.

## Source

Department of Human Biology, NUTRIM School for Nutrition, Toxicology and Metabolism, Maastricht University Medical Centre+ (MUMC+), Maastricht, Netherlands.

## Abstract

In recent years, it has been shown that humans have active brown adipose tissue (BAT) depots, raising the question of whether activation and recruitment of BAT can be a target to counterbalance the current obesity pandemic. Here, we show that a 10-day cold acclimation protocol in humans increases BAT activity in parallel with an increase in nonshivering thermogenesis (NST). No sex differences in BAT presence and activity were found either before or after cold acclimation. Respiration measurements in permeabilized fibers and isolated mitochondria revealed no significant contribution of skeletal muscle mitochondrial uncoupling to the increased NST. Based on cell-specific markers and on uncoupling protein-1 (characteristic of both BAT and beige/brite cells), this study did not show "browning" of abdominal subcutaneous white adipose tissue upon cold acclimation. The observed physiological acclimation is in line with the subjective changes in temperature sensation; upon cold acclimation, the subjects judged the environment warmer, felt more comfortable in the cold, and reported less shivering. The combined results suggest that a variable indoor environment with frequent cold exposures might be an acceptable and economic manner to increase energy expenditure and may contribute to counteracting the current obesity epidemic.

Comment in Obesity: Cold Exposure Increases Brown Adipose Tissue in Humans [*Nat Rev Endocrinol.* 2013].

Obesity: Cold Exposure Increases Brown Adipose Tissue in Humans. *Greenhill C. Nat Rev Endocrinol. 2013 Oct; 9(10):566. Epub 2013 Aug 6.*

PMID: 23867626

# Brown Fat Activation Mediates Cold-Induced Thermogenesis in Adult Humans in Response to a Mild Decrease in Ambient Temperature

Chen, K.Y., R. J. Brychta, J. D. Linderman, S. Smith, A. Courville, W. Dieckmann, P. Herscovitch, C. M. Millo, A. Remaley, P. Lee, and F. S. Celi. *J Clin Endocrinol Metab.* 98 no. 7 (July 2013): E1218-23. doi: 10.1210/jc.2012-4213. Epub June 18, 2013.

## Source

Diabetes, Endocrinology, and Obesity Branch, National Institute of Diabetes and Digestive and Kidney Diseases, Clinical Center, National Institutes of Health, Bethesda, Maryland 20892-1613, USA.

## Abstract

Context:

The contribution of brown adipose tissue (BAT) to the energy balance in humans exposed to sustainable cold has not been completely established, partially because of measurement limitations of both BAT activity and energy expenditure (EE).

Objective:

The objective of the study was to characterize the role of BAT activation in cold-induced thermogenesis (CIT).

Design:

This study was a single-blind, randomized crossover intervention.

Setting:

The study was conducted at the National Institutes of Health Clinical Center.

Study Participants:

Thirty-one healthy volunteers participated in the study.

Interventions:

The intervention included mild cold exposure.

Main Outcomes:

CIT and BAT activation were the main outcomes in this study.

Methods:

Overnight EE measurement by whole-room indirect calo-
rimeter at 24 °C or 19 °C was followed by 2-[18F]-fluoro-
2-deoxy-D-glucose positron emission tomography (PET)
scan. After 36 hours, volunteers crossed over to the
alternate study temperature under identical conditions.
BAT activity was measured in a 3-dimensional region of
interest in the upper torso by comparing the uptake at the
two temperatures.

Results:

Twenty-four volunteers (14 males, 10 females) had a
complete data set. When compared with 24 °C, exposure
at 19 °C resulted in increased EE (5.3 ± 5.9%, P < .001),
indicating CIT response and mean BAT activity (10.5 ±
11.1%, P < .001). Multiple regression analysis indicated
that a difference in BAT activity (P < .001), age (P = .01),
and gender (P = .037) were independent contributors to
individual variability of CIT.

Conclusions:

A small reduction in ambient temperature, within the
range of climate-controlled buildings, is sufficient to
increase human BAT activity, which correlates with

individual CIT response. This study uncovers for the first time a spectrum of BAT activation among healthy adults during mild cold exposure not previously recognized by conventional PET and PET-computed tomography methods. The enhancement of cold-induced BAT stimulation may represent a novel environmental strategy in obesity treatment.

PMID: 23780370

## BMP7 Activates Brown Adipose Tissue and Reduces Diet-Induced Obesity Only at Subthermoneutrality

Boon, M.R., S. A. van den Berg, Y. Wang, J. van den Bossche, S. Karkampouna, M. Bauwens, M. De Saint-Hubert, G. van der Horst, S. Vukicevic, M. P. de Winther, L. M. Havekes, J. W. Jukema, J. T. Tamsma, G. van der Pluijm, K. W. van Dijk, and P. C. Rensen. *PLoS One.* 2013 Sep 16;8(9):e74083. doi: 10.1371/journal.pone.0074083.

## Source

Department of Endocrinology and Metabolic Diseases, Leiden University Medical Center, Leiden, The Netherlands; Einthoven Laboratory for Experimental Vascular Medicine, Leiden University Medical Center, Leiden, The Netherlands.

## Abstract

Background/Aims:

Brown adipose tissue (BAT) dissipates energy stored in triglycerides as heat via the uncoupling protein UCP-1 and is a promising target to combat hyperlipidemia and obesity. BAT is densely innervated by the sympathetic nervous system, which increases BAT differentiation and activity upon cold exposure. Recently, Bone Morphogenetic Protein 7 (BMP7) was identified as an inducer of BAT differentiation. We aimed to elucidate the role of sympathetic activation in the effect of BMP7 on BAT by treating mice with BMP7 at varying ambient temperature, and assessed the therapeutic potential of BMP7 in combating obesity.

Methods and Results:

High-fat diet fed lean C57Bl6/J mice were treated with BMP7 via subcutaneous osmotic minipumps for 4 weeks at 21°C or 28°C, the latter being a thermoneutral temperature in which sympathetic activation of BAT is largely diminished. At 21°C, BMP7 increased BAT weight, increased the expression of Ucp1, Cd36 and hormone-sensitive lipase in BAT, and increased total energy expenditure. BMP7 treatment markedly increased food intake without affecting physical activity. Despite that, BMP7 diminished white adipose tissue (WAT) mass, accompanied by increased expression of genes related to intracellular lipolysis in WAT. All these effects were blunted at 28°C. Additionally, BMP7 resulted in extensive "browning" of WAT, as evidenced by increased expression of BAT markers and the appearance of whole clusters of brown adipocytes via immunohistochemistry, independent of environmental temperature. Treatment of diet-induced obese C57Bl6/J mice with BMP7 led to an improved metabolic phenotype, consisting of a decreased fat mass and liver lipids as well as attenuated dyslipidemia and hyperglycemia.

Conclusion:

Together, these data show that BMP7-mediated recruitment and activation of BAT only occurs at subthermoneutral temperature, and is thus likely dependent on sympathetic activation of BAT, and that BMP7 may be a promising tool to combat obesity and associated disorders.

PMID: 24066098

**Could Increased Time Spent in a Thermal Comfort Zone Contribute to Population Increases in Obesity?**

versity College London, London, UK.

## Abstract

Domestic winter indoor temperatures in the USA, UK and other developed countries appear to be following an upwards trend. This review examines evidence of a causal link between thermal exposures and increases in obesity prevalence, focusing on acute and longer-term biological effects of time spent in thermal comfort compared with mild cold. Reduced exposure to seasonal cold may have a dual effect on energy expenditure, both minimizing the need for physiological thermogenesis and reducing thermogenic capacity. Experimental studies show a graded association between acute mild cold and human energy expenditure over the range of temperatures relevant to indoor heating trends. Meanwhile, recent studies of the role of brown adipose tissue (BAT) in human thermogenesis suggest that increased time spent in conditions of thermal comfort can lead to a loss of BAT and reduced thermogenic capacity. Pathways linking cold exposure and adiposity have not been directly tested in humans. Research in naturalistic and experimental settings is needed to establish effects of changes in thermal exposures on weight, which may raise possibilities for novel public health strategies to address obesity.

PMID: 21261804

## Cold Prevents the Light-Induced Inactivation of Pineal N-Acetyltransferase in the Djungarian Hamster, Phodopus Sungorus

Stieglitz, A., S. Steinlechner, T. Ruf, G. Heldmaier. *J Comp Physiol A*. 168 no. 5 (May 1991):599–603.

## Source

Department of Biology/Zoology, Philipps-University, Marburg, Germany

## Abstract

In the Djungarian hamster seasonal acclimatization is primarily controlled by photoperiod, but exposure to low ambient temperature amplifies the intensity and duration of short day-induced winter adaptations. The aim of this study was to test, whether the pineal gland is involved in integrating both environmental cues. Exposure of hamsters to cold (0 degrees C) reduces the sensitivity of the pineal gland to light at night and prevents inactivation of N-acetyltransferase (NAT). The parallel time course of NAT activity and plasma norepinephrine content suggests that circulating catecholamines may stimulate melatonin synthesis under cold load.

PMID: 1920160

## Diurnal Changes in Sensitivity to Melatonin in Intact and Pinealectomized Djungarian Hamsters: Effects on Thermogenesis, Cold Tolerance, and Gonads

Holtorf, A. P., G. Heldmaier, G. Thiele, S. Steinlechner. *J Pineal Res.* 2 no. 4 (1985): 393–403.

## Abstract

Djungarian hamsters kept in long photoperiod (16:8 L:D) were injected daily at 0800, 1200, or 1600 with 25 micrograms of melatonin. During 90 days of treatment, body weight and fur coloration were checked at weekly intervals, and at the end of the treatment the reproductive

status of the hamsters and their thermoregulatory properties (could limit, maximum thermoregulatory heat production, nonshivering thermogenesis, cytochrome oxidase
activity in brown adipose tissue) were measured. Hamsters injected at 1600 changed from summer to winter
status with regard to all functions investigated respond-
ing simultaneously; i.e., their body weights decreased,
their fur became white, their gonads regressed, and their
thermoregulatory properties improved. All these changes
were identical to the effects of short photoperiod (8:16
L:D) exposure. Injections of melatonin at 0800 and 1200
were ineffective for reproductive functions, but the injection of melatonin at 0800 caused slight improvements
of thermogenesis. The response to melatonin injected
at 1600 could be suppressed by an additional injection
of melatonin at 0800 (75 micrograms). Pinealectomized
or ganglionectomized hamsters kept in long photoperiod
did not respond to daily injections of melatonin at 1600
for the first 60 days of treatment, but during a prolonged
treatment their sensitivity to melatonin was restored. Sim-
ilarly, pinealectomized or ganglionectomized hamsters
failed to respond to short photoperiod for about 40 days,
but during prolonged exposure their sensitivity to short
photoperiod was restored.

PMID: 3831320

This paper from 1981 shows that short days and melatonin have the same positive effect on brown fat production. We need low-blue-light glasses for hamsters.

## Photoperiodic Control and Effects of Melatonin on Nonshivering Thermogenesis and Brown Adipose Tissue

Heldmaier, G., S. Steinlechner, J. Rafael, P. Vsiansky. *Science* 212 (4497) (May 22, 1981): 917–9.

## Abstract

Exposure to a short photoperiod improved the thermogenic capacity, and cold resistance of Djungarian hamsters and increased the respiratory power of their brown adipose tissue. Exposure to a long photoperiod caused a decrease in thermogenic measurements. This thermotropic action of the short photoperiod was detectable only during late summer and fall. A similar thermotropic response could be elicited by implanting hamsters with melatonin, indicating that the pineal may be involved in photoperiodic control of thermoregulatory effectors.

PMID: 7233183

# CHAPTER 9
## Other Ways That Light Affects Health

Controlling light to improve sleep goes a long way to improving health. Avoiding a disruption of the circadian rhythm helps maintain good mental health. Maximizing melatonin is the other aspect of how controlling light plays an important role in avoiding illness. For a discussion of some of the benefits of maximizing melatonin, a few press releases issued over the past few years are used in part of the following.

## Breast Cancer, Colon Cancer, and Prostate Cancer

I am confident that maximizing melatonin by use of our products will also reduce the risk of at least the cancers that are stimulated by estrogen (most breast cancer and prostate cancer). However, until clinical trials have shown a consistent benefit, the FDA rules do not permit making such claims. Fortunately, the average person can draw his or her own conclusions and take appropriate action to guard his or her own health.

A lot of our awareness of the importance of maximizing melatonin is the result of a series of studies by Dr. Eva Schernhammer at

Women's Hospital, part of the Harvard School of Medicine. Her 2001 paper observed that nurses who had worked night shift for many years had a significantly higher incidence of breast cancer than those who had not worked night shift. It offered evidence that the melatonin hypothesis was correct. The so-called melatonin hypothesis (Stevens 1996) postulates that the increased risk in breast cancer in recent decades in industrialized countries results in part from increased exposure to light at night[5]. A later study by Schernhammer and others found the same situation with colon cancer. As with breast cancer, nurses who had worked the night shift for many years had a higher incidence. Many studies in animals have shown that long nights (i.e., fourteen hours of darkness) resulted in reduced incidences of breast cancer compared to eight hours of darkness (as most humans experience).

Several years ago, based on the evidence that working the night shift increased the incidence of breast cancer, the Danish government provided financial compensation to thirty-eight nurses who had worked the night shift for a number of years and subsequently developed breast cancer. There is a second theory that it is the disruption of the circadian cycle as a result of shiftwork that increases the risk of breast cancer rather than the reduction in the amount of melatonin produced. In either case, using amber glasses or special light bulbs may be a way to avoid an increased risk of breast and other cancers.

---

[5] Environ Health Perspect. 1996 Mar;104 Suppl 1:135-40.
**The melatonin hypothesis: electric power and breast cancer.**
Stevens RG, Davis S.

Prostate cancer is also elevated in night-shift workers compared to day-shift workers. Again, there are the two theories, disruption of the circadian rhythm and suppression of melatonin. Controlling light with special light bulbs or amber glasses may help one avoid both of the suspected causes of the increase in prostate cancer in night-shift workers.

## Metastasis of Cancer

Metastasis of cancer to distant sites is the thing that kills most cancer patients, not the original tumor. A breakthrough study[6] at Tulane and Thomas Jefferson Medical Schools showed that the increased risk of metastasis of both breast cancer and prostate cancer can result from disrupting the circadian (daily) cycle causing loss of melatonin due to exposure to light at night. Avoiding the blue rays in ordinary white light for four hours before bedtime, coupled with eight hours of sleep in darkness, may restore the full twelve hours of melatonin flow known to be possible.

The study examined the molecular processes involved in the transition of stable cancer cells into cancer cells capable of moving through the bloodstream to distant sites where new tumors can develop. They examined how the presence of various compounds

---

[6] J Pineal Res. 2011 Oct;51(3):259-69. doi: 10.1111/j.1600-079X.2011.00888.x. Epub 2011 May 24.
Circadian regulation of molecular, dietary, and metabolic signaling mechanisms of human breast cancer growth by the nocturnal melatonin signal and the consequences of its disruption by light at night.
Blask DE, Hill SM, Dauchy RT, Xiang S, Yuan L, Duplessis T, Mao L, Dauchy E, Sauer LA.

required for the different steps in the process were associated with the presence or absence of melatonin. They looked at this in both cultured cancer cells (breast cancer and prostate cancer) and human cancers grown as grafts on the backs of rats but supplied with human blood. In every case, cancer cells retained a static structure when melatonin was present; however, in the absence of melatonin, the conditions necessary for metastasis to occur were observed. The blood without melatonin was obtained from volunteers either during the day or during the night after two-hour exposure to bright light. The blood with melatonin was from volunteers either during the night when they were kept in darkness or during the day following oral administration of a melatonin supplement.

The transition of the cancer cells from one type to the other is a complex process. Reducing the risk of metastasis is not complex or difficult. A study at the University of Toronto seven years ago found that blocking blue light (wavelength less than about 530 nanometers) with amber eyeglasses restored melatonin as if the subjects were in darkness even though they were exposed to bright lights during the night. Such glasses, along with light bulbs that don't produce blue light and filters for TVs, tablets, and smartphones are available at lowbluelights.com.

## Seasonal Affective Disorder (SAD)

The standard treatment for seasonal affective disorder (SAD) or the winter blues is to expose the eyes to bright light for about a half an hour first thing in the morning. This has been demonstrated to advance the start of the flow of melatonin to an earlier hour. By starting earlier, it finishes its flow earlier. Thus solves the problem of too much melatonin in the morning. For some people, the idea of sitting in front of a bright light first thing in the morning is unpleasant and simply not practical. There is also concern it might damage the eyes (macular degeneration).

In 2001, it was discovered that the flow of melatonin is controlled primarily by the exposure of the eyes to blue light or the blue rays in ordinary white light. Most modern light boxes used to treat SAD use blue light. Exposing the eyes to light in the evening prevents the flow of melatonin from starting. Wearing glasses that block blue light allows the flow to start. The average time for melatonin to flow (if the person is in darkness) is 11.4 hours, according to a recent study[7]. Putting on glasses at 7:00 p.m. should allow the flow to be over by 7:00 a.m. With melatonin gone, you may wake up feeling happy, without the need for an alarm clock. Because the glasses only block blue light, there is plenty of light by which to read or carry on normal evening activities. For those who don't like to wear glasses, low-blue-light light bulbs are available, as are filters for tablets, smartphones, and other screens.

---

[7] PLoS One. 2008 Aug 26;3(8):e3055. doi: 10.1371/journal.pone.0003055.
**Individual differences in the amount and timing of salivary melatonin secretion.**
Burgess HJ, Fogg LF.

# Alzheimer's Disease

In recent papers from Italy, Russia, and the United States, scientists have described the possible benefits of melatonin in avoiding and treating Alzheimer's disease. Wearing special glasses that block the blue light known to suppress melatonin allows it to flow as if in darkness. In this way, the glasses available at lowbluelights. com allow the body to produce melatonin for eleven to twelve hours. Because of exposure to light in the hours before bedtime, most people only make melatonin for seven or eight hours a night.

A recent study of the spinal fluid that bathes the brain suggests this difference in the time that the pineal gland makes melatonin (and other antioxidants) may affect the probability for the formation of the plaques associated with Alzheimer's disease. Studies in animals and humans show that the concentration of melatonin in the spinal fluid is significantly higher than in the blood. Melatonin is thought to be the unique antioxidant that protects the brain from damage by eliminating the free radicals that can damage the brain cells.

# Attention Deficit Hyperactivity Disorder (ADHD)

Adults with attention deficit hyperactivity disorder (ADHD) and insomnia experienced significant improvement in measurements of overall sleep quality with the use of glasses that block blue light, according to Dr. Fargason, author of a paper submitted to the journal (and provided to this author) *ChronoPhysiology Therapy*.

"Compared to baseline, the intervention resulted in significant improvement in global PSQI (Pittsburg Sleep Quality Index) scores, PSQI subcomponent scores, and sleep diary measures of morning refreshment after sleep (P = 0.0377) and nighttime awakenings (P = 0.015). Global PSQI scores fell from 11.15 to 4.54, dropping below the cut-off score for clinical insomnia," wrote Dr. Fargason.

Twenty-four people (ages twenty-one to seventy-six, mean age 43.9 years) began the three-month study, but only fourteen completed it. This is not surprising in light of the nature of attention deficit hyperactivity disorder, according to Dr. Richard Hansler, who led the group at John Carroll University that developed the glasses in 2005. He further commented, "Use of light bulbs that eliminate blue light and filters for TV, computer screens and for phones, might be a way of achieving higher compliance in future tests. Many people who do not normally wear glasses may find it difficult to wear them in the evening." Of the fourteen subjects who completed the test, the seven with the latest bedtime experienced an advance to an earlier hour of their bedtime of an average of forty-three minutes.

The blue-light-blocking glasses for this study were donated by Photonic Developments. They also provide light bulbs that eliminate blue light and filters for TV, computer, tablet, and smartphone screens. These products were developed in 2005 in the Lighting Innovations Institute at John Carroll University.

## Type 2 Diabetes

Nurses with the highest melatonin production have about half the type 2 diabetes of those with the lowest melatonin, according to the Harvard study. Orange eyeglasses that eliminate blue light (available from Photonic Developments LLC) help maximize melatonin production.

In the April 3, 2013, issue of the *Journal of the American Medical Association* scientists from the Harvard School of Public Health describe the results of a thirteen-year study of the incidence of type 2 diabetes in nurses participating in the Nurses' Health Study. Quoting from the abstract, "Among participants without diabetes who provided urine and blood samples at baseline in 2000, we identified 370 women who developed type 2 diabetes from 2000–2012 and matched 370 controls using risk-set sampling. Associations between melatonin secretion at baseline and incidence of type 2 diabetes were evaluated with multivariable conditional logistic regression controlling for demographic characteristics, lifestyle habits, measures of sleep quality..." Comparing the results they found, "Women in the highest category of melatonin secretion had an estimated diabetes incidence rate of 4.27 cases/1000 person-years compared with 9.27 cases/1000 person-years in the lowest category." That is, those with the highest melatonin were less than half as likely to develop type 2 diabetes as those in the lowest melatonin category.

A study in 2005 conducted at the University of Toronto found that wearing orange goggles that blocked the blue part of the spectrum out to a wavelength of about 530 nanometers allowed the subjects to produce melatonin during the night just as they had when kept in darkness, despite being exposed to bright lights. Based upon this and several animal studies, a group of physicists at John Carroll University developed light bulbs that don't produce blue light and eyeglasses that eliminate it as well as filters for TV and computer screens and even for tablets and smartphones. They are sold by Photonic Developments LLC at www.lowbluelights.com. Most people buy the company's products to help them sleep better. There is a money-back guarantee if a customer's sleep does not improve. The possible reduction in the risk of type 2 diabetes is a free bonus. Nearly 90 percent of the customers who try these products find they improve their sleep. Many find success after years of trying practically everything else.

## Bipolar Disorder

### Dark Therapy for Bipolar Disorder Using Amber Lenses for Blue Light Blockade

Phelps, J. Med Hypotheses 70 no. 2 (2008): 224–9. Epub, July 16, 2007.

Richard L. Hansler, PhD

## Source

Corvallis Psychiatric Clinic, 3517 Samaritan Drive, Corvallis, OR 97330, United States.

## Abstract

"Dark Therapy", in which complete darkness is used as a mood stabilizer in bipolar disorder, roughly the converse of light therapy for depression, has support in several preliminary studies. Although data are limited, darkness itself appears to organize and stabilize circadian rhythms. Yet insuring complete darkness from 6 p.m. to 8 a.m. the following morning, as used in several studies thus far, is highly impractical and not accepted by patients. However, recent data on the physiology of human circadian rhythm suggests that "virtual darkness" may be achievable by blocking blue wavelengths of light. A recently discovered retinal photoreceptor, whose fibers connect only to the biological clock region of the hypothalamus, has been shown to respond only to a narrow band of wavelengths around 450 nm. Amber-tinted safety glasses, which block transmission of these wavelengths, have already been shown to preserve normal nocturnal melatonin levels in a light environment which otherwise completely suppresses melatonin production. Therefore it may be possible to influence human circadian rhythms by using these lenses at night to blunt the impact of electrical light, particularly the blue light of ubiquitous television screens, by creating a "virtual darkness". One way to investigate this would be to provide the lenses to patients with severe sleep disturbance of probable circadian origin. A preliminary case series herein demonstrates that some patients with bipolar disorder experience reduced sleep-onset latency with this approach, suggesting a circadian effect. If amber lenses can effectively simulate darkness, a broad range of conditions might respond to this inexpensive therapeutic tool: common forms of insomnia; **sleep deprivation in nursing mothers**; circadian rhythm disruption in shift workers; and perhaps even rapid cycling bipolar disorder, a difficult-to-treat variation of a common illness.

If you are reading this you have earned my thanks for going the distance. I'll end this book the same as I've ended earlier ones with the simple statement that "Without action, knowledge has little value"

Made in the USA
Charleston, SC
25 February 2014